MY ANGEL TREE

MY ANGEL TREE

In Loving Memory of My Dear Daughter

Jessica Alice Leigh-Firbank

25th May 1990 - 18th February 2002

*"I'll love you forever and know you to be
An Angel in Heaven but a part of Me"*

Kirsty Bilski

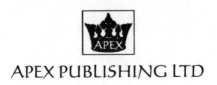

APEX PUBLISHING LTD

First published in 2008 by

Apex Publishing Ltd

PO Box 7086, Clacton on Sea, Essex, CO15 5WN

www.apexpublishing.co.uk

British Library Cataloguing-in-Publication Data
A catalogue record for this book
is available from the British Library

ISBN 1-906358-10-9   978-1-906358-10-5

Typeset in 10.5pt Bskerville Win95BT

Production Manager: Chris Cowlin

Cover Design: Siobhan Smith

Printed and bound by Biddles Ltd.,
Kings Lynn, Norfolk

A huge thank you and much love to Jerzy, Gemma and Stewart for enabling completion of this book and for believing in me.

A special thanks also to all the professionals who dedicated so much time to helping Jess and continue in their commitment to support other children and their families:

Children's Hospice South West: www.chsw.org.uk
CLIC Sargent: www.clicsargent.org.uk
The Make-a-Wish Foundation: www.make-a-wish.org.uk
The Rainbow Centre: www.rainbowcentre.org.uk
BIBIC: www.bibic.org.uk
The Children's Unit, Musgrove Park Hospital, Taunton
Bristol Royal Hospital for Children
Birmingham Children's Hospital

Foreword

I first became involved with Children's Hospice South West over 15 years ago in the run up to the opening of Little Bridge House. I am to this day extremely proud to be patron of such a wonderful organisation. I particularly remember one young man usually confined to a wheelchair, who was thrilled to join me in my helicopter for a short flight. It was when he said in answer to my question 'Have you enjoyed the flight?' - 'Yes, particularly when I was able to look down on my wheelchair' that I first realised that I was going to learn more from these young people who face up to death at such an early age than I could ever give in return.

I always had a standing joke with the founder Jill Farwell that she must never thank me for my visits. I told her that I should be the one saying 'thank you' because I am the one who gains so much from spending time with the children and meeting their families.

People often tell me they would rather run a mile than visit a children's hospice, they fear that it will be depressing, bleak and full of sick children suffering in their beds. The reality is that it is not depressing, but uplifting. A child's life might be short, but they live each day with courage and to the full, so the hospice rings with life and laughter and although there is sadness, it is sadness shared and the power of love, courage, and friendship shines through. This may be difficult to believe, but if you read My Angel Tree, Kirsty Bilski's moving tribute to her daughter Jess, it will help you understand.

On the face of it you may feel My Angel Tree offers bleak reading - for it is Kirsty's account of her eldest daughter's diagnosis with liver cancer, the illness and treatments endured, and the sad and untimely death of Jess at the age of 11 years. But the success of the book, and its very essence, is that this unbearably sad experience is transformed into an uplifting and heart warming story.

With the consummate skill of an eloquent and articulate writer, coupled with the wisdom and insight of a mother who has suffered one of life's hardest blows, Kirsty takes the reader by the hand and draws them step by step along the journey the family took with Jess. As we travel this road we witness heartbreak, pain, loss and anguish, but more importantly we share immense fortitude, enduring love, a strong faith and the spirit of family - so that in the end we draw courage, inspiration and hope from this deeply moving story.

Sadly, I never met Jess. She came to the hospice when she was very ill and, although I had made arrangements to meet her at Little Bridge House, she died before the visit could take place. It is particularly poignant, therefore, that her mother has brought Jess so vividly to life on the pages of her book. Jess's story will inspire you with her valiant fight for life and move you as she faces up to death with a maturity beyond her years, and we all have the privilege of getting to know Jess in a way I wish I had been able to do during her life.

On one of my very first visits to Little Bridge House I met a mum who was staying alongside her son who was in the last weeks of his life. We spoke at length and her words touched my heart and have stayed with me ever since. Although, like Kirsty, she was facing the tragedy of her child's premature death she told me: 'The one thing we have learnt is that love is stronger than death'. Kirsty Bilski's book is living proof of this and if you would like to reaffirm your belief in the resilience of the human spirit and the strength of family, then I urge you to read this story – it will remind you of what lies at the heart of our humanity.

Noel Edmonds

Introduction

The twenty-fifth of May would have been her eighteenth birthday. I wonder how we would have celebrated; I'm sure we would have had a party. I know the laughter and fun we would have enjoyed together. I close my eyes and I see every detail of her face as it was back then - I knew it so well - and yet I wonder how she might look now, had life given her a chance. I remember the sparkle in her bright blue eyes as she smiled up at me. Her hearty sense of humour and that dimple, so characteristic of her cheery expression. She possessed an inner beauty, generosity of spirit and a warm heart.

It's been more than six years since she left us. She didn't want to go, but she came to know her future as being in a different place; close enough to still be a part of our lives, but distance would be inevitable. Her faith formed visions of how her existence would continue. We talked together of warmth, colour and light; a place where there would be no more pain. She didn't want to die, but she couldn't face the treatment anymore. She courageously accepted the truth of her decline and suffered both physical and psychological pain as she battled through those last few months.

The memories of our time together will live with me always. She was more than just a daughter, she was my friend and we shared so much. I feel so proud to have been her mum and blessed to have loved such a special child. She was intelligent and humorous. She loved life, valued her friends and cared deeply about her family. Losing her tore me apart, with a pain that reached to the very depths of my soul. It has been hard to carry on without her, but my two remaining children guide the way for me. I see echoes of her in them, reminding me of her spirit and helping me to reach for the future.

My life has not been an easily travelled road, but through everything I have unconditionally loved all three of my children, each completing my world in their own individual ways. Should any one of them have been taken from me, my pain would have been equal. I hope one day my younger two will read this book and know their sister a little better, perhaps learning about me too. As a mum who chose to allow honesty to guide my heart, I shared everything that happened with my children. It is my hope that the words in this book will help them to remember other special moments of their own.

I began writing as a gift to Gemma and Stewart, a way of remembering a special sister who loved them dearly. But, along the way, it became a therapeutic space for me, where I could lose myself in memories and never quite let go. I had tried to finish it often, but experienced a sense of being stuck, not just in writing but in life as well. In being lost, the book became my journey home. I came to recognise that its completion would represent a final acceptance in me; a way of holding her close but accepting that she was finally gone and knowing peace again.

After she died I found a diary in which she had written that she wanted to be a teacher when she grew up. I believe she had already achieved this: she taught so much to so many, those who knew her personally and those who only came to hear of her courage - she touched people's hearts and changed lives. To know her story is the gift of an experience where both learning and reassurance can be found. It is my hope that through the pages of this book she will continue to reach out in the future, like the branches of a tree reaching towards the sunlight, providing both shade and comfort to those in need. And now it is complete my journey home is done and new possibilities open up to me. But at the heart of my future she will always be my truest inspiration. And so through the enormity of this completition, just as my darling daughter I have now also found peace.

Kirsty Bilski
September 2008

Chapter 1

Through the slightly open window I could hear the distant chatter of voices: my guests had started to arrive. It was a beautiful day and the sun shone brightly, only occasionally obscured by wispy white clouds, glorious gold reflecting on the last of the spring daffodils. Nobody seemed to notice the slight chill in the air. Torrential rain over the past few days had threatened to overshadow our time, but the brightness of this morning refreshed our spirits. The picturesque gardens of this stony old mill provided the perfect setting. The millstream twisted and splashed a course down the gentle slope and finally tumbled into a fresh, sparkling pool. Watery sounds travelled on the cool spring breeze, a gentle background trickle of calm and reassurance reaching out to welcome guests as they gradually gathered. I nervously got myself ready. I could vaguely make out the voice of my husband-to-be partaking of polite conversation with various family members. I listened intently. He sounded nervous and a little worse for wear after having enjoyed a few drinks too many with friends the night before. If he was feeling a little fragile, it was totally self-inflicted.

More and more of our family were arriving and there were now so many people chattering that individual voices were disguised. I looked at myself in the mirror, admiring my elegant, long, satin and lace dress. I had asked for something simple but, in her usual style, Mum had created a dress fit for a 'princess'. My personal reflection fell somewhat short of this description, but I felt wonderful, high on the adrenalin of the occasion and totally in love. A nervous excitement had grown in me for weeks now and today would be the culmination of all the planning but, most importantly, a reflection of the hopes and dreams we shared together.

My hands were shaking as I applied the finishing touches to my make-up. I was feeling quite nervous now but certainly not unsure. My past had been a difficult journey, but Jerzy had gradually and gently gained my trust, changing not just my life

1

but the lives of my children completely, and the sadness of previous memories had gradually faded away as our love grew and united us as a new family.

An antique clock ornately revealed that there were just ten minutes to go. I sipped the last of my complimentary brandy whilst taking a final look in the mirror, before quietly leaving my room in search of my brother. He was already on his way downstairs and we continued out into the sunshine together. I stepped out squinting, as I had not been prepared for such a vast contrast in the quality of the light. Cathy was anxiously waiting for us outside, ready with her camera to capture this very special day. As the daughter of Jerzy's previous partner, Annie, I was proud that our friendship had led to this kind gesture on her part. As her camera clicked busily we moved closer to the marriage room, which lay up a flight of sweeping stone steps at the end of the building. There was an unnatural hush now. All my guests were obviously seated and waiting for me to appear. As I tried gracefully to climb the steps, I was met by a whole host of excited children.

Firstly there was my niece and god-daughter, Alice. She was not yet two years old but certainly understood the excitement of the occasion and looked adorable in her matching green and cream satin organza dress. Then there were Ellie, Sammy, Katie and Hannah. Being the daughters of my closest friend, Sarah, they had grown up alongside my children. When they accepted the responsibility of being bridesmaids I couldn't have been more delighted. Sarah and I had met when Hannah and my eldest daughter, Jessica, were very small babies. Aged only six weeks apart they shared much of their childhood together. Now they were both ten years old and, on reflection, time had seemed to flash by. Sarah and her family were a huge part of my world, and the importance to me of their involvement in the day's proceedings could never be adequately expressed in words.

As I continued up the steps my youngest, Stewart, stepped forward and clung to my hand. Being just five years old, he was pleased at last to find me and anxious not to let go. Stasia, Jerzy's niece, was the next one to greet me. The same age as Hannah and Jess, Stasia completed the chattering trio who could regularly be found immersed in the latest music and fashion together. Then bouncing towards me came Gemma, my middle daughter, who was clearly tremendously excited and was finding it hard to contain a bubbly feeling that made her bob up and down uncontrollably. She looked an absolute picture, and the smile on her face and glint in her eye expressed a thousand unspoken words. She took a deep breath and gave me an enormous hug. Gemma was the free spirit of the family and acted as her emotions dictated, often finding herself in a tough place, but no amount of persuasion could ever change her direction. She seemed to learn best from making her own mistakes even at this young age, a quality I admired and a strength that would help her to surf the stormy seas of life.

Finally, after finding my way through these children, I found my Jess, a vision etched into my memory in such detail to this day. Her hair shone healthily, matching the glow in her cheeks, and her eyes sparkled with tears of joy. The honesty in her smile revealed an otherwise hidden dimple, which had no hope of disappearing for hours yet. She suddenly seemed so grown up, standing taller than the other girls and proudly wearing her matching dress, As chief bridesmaid she took her responsibility very seriously. Jess had many wonderful qualities; amongst many others she was kind, thoughtful and valued everyone. She used her intelligence to give confidence and encouragement to others, often reaching out to teach or guide her peers where she could. As I watched her this day, I truly understood her natural beauty. She had the power to light up a room with honesty and grace, a rare and sensitive gift. She filled me with pride.

I stood for a second and drank in the wonder of the moment. The children were all chattering excitedly, trying not to make too much noise as they waited to begin this wonderful day. I hugged Jess and returned to the back of the queue, leaving her proudly to lead the way through the centre aisle of this atmospheric old room.

Just as they had rehearsed, the children stepped away in turn, their heads bobbing up and down and mirroring the tempo of the music. For the first time that day, I caught sight of Jerzy, who was looking past the children and straight at me. On catching his gaze my nerves melted away; inwardly I knew everything

3

was going to be fine. As he stood patiently waiting for me to join him, I noticed that his complexion was glowing too. I hoped it was due in part to the love he felt for me, although in truth the events of the night before could have had something to do with it!

Alice followed on behind the girls as they stepped through the middle of our guests, but she very soon lost momentum and drifted, causing an obstruction in the middle of the aisle. She captured everyone's attention, laughter crept across the faces of her audience and she clearly enjoyed being centre stage! Unfortunately, this unscripted behaviour meant that Kevin, Stewart and I couldn't get through. It seemed to take an age to get to Jerzy, perhaps more because of my eagerness than because of Alice's inquisitiveness towards her audience, but we got there in the end. I was so pleased finally to make it that I forgot to hand Jess my flowers. She reminded me quite abruptly as if to awaken me from a dream. I admired the responsible way in which she had taken it upon herself to make sure that my bouquet was suitably cared for - so typical of my eldest child to mother everyone, including me!

Jerzy and I had put a lot of time into planning the service. We had arranged for a civil ceremony led by the local Registrar, who married us in a little over ten minutes! That was fine, however, as we had wanted to attach more importance to the blessing, which followed straight afterwards and was led by the vicar of Bicknoller, the Reverend Alfrida Savigear. Our faith was a strong part of our relationship and, although we were not to marry in church, we had wanted our beliefs to be included in our ceremony. The children introduced the blessing with a song they all knew from school, although they sang much quieter than they had in our rehearsal. I think the younger ones amongst them had not realised that there would be 'people' there! The ceremony went exactly as we had planned and the involvement of the children all the way through meant a huge amount to both of us. As we prepared to bring the service to an end, Jess took her turn. She had prepared a poem called 'The Gift of Lasting Love' by Helen Steiner Rice. She stepped forward, looked at me for encouragement and then proceeded to read. She had been determined to read a poem: this day,

4

Jerzy, our love and her family were of the utmost importance to her and this was her way of showing that to everyone. With such poise, courage and determination, she spoke these words:

Love is much more than a tender caress
And more than bright hours of gay happiness
For a lasting love is made up of sharing
Both hours that are Joyous and also Despairing
It's made up of patience and deep understanding
And never of selfish and stubborn demanding
It's made up of climbing the steep hills together
And facing with courage life's stormiest weather
Nothing on earth or in heaven can part
A love that has grown part of the heart
Just like the sun and the stars and the sea
This love will go on through eternity
For true love lives on when earthly things die
*For it's part of the spirit that soars to the sky.**

* *Used with permission of The Helen Steiner Rice Foundation, Cincinnati, Ohio.*

These words have come to hold another meaning for me now. How could we have known then how closely they might come to reflect our future? I have since found comfort here in the knowledge that Jess believed that death wasn't final and the spirit would live on. We often spoke about love. She believed that we don't leave this earth with nothing; we take the love of our friends and family with us to a special place. Whether that be heaven or a spirit world, Jess believed that there was more and that love was the key.

Finally we walked out again into the glorious sunshine, 'Morning Has Broken' playing gently in the background. I felt as though everything was so perfect and nothing could possibly ever change. Immediately after the service, Jess found me. Although tearful, she assured me that nothing was wrong. She just wanted me to know how much she loved us all. She was overwhelmed by the occasion and deliriously happy. She had found it difficult to contain herself, but once she had shared this and hugged us both she was soon running around with her friends again. The rest of this day is a glorious memory of laughter and fun: a perfectly beautiful reception; a marquee filled with balloons, which the children soon dismantled, before weaving excitedly between the tables clutching huge bunches of colour. We had a clown, who entertained everyone, not just the children. He also managed to get us up dancing, Sarah somehow ended up on the floor waggling her legs in the air! He did a few choice magic tricks but found it hard to fool the children and particularly Jess, who seemed to have all the answers. The spirit of the occasion drifted on well into the night. What a day, such a glorious day, and one that I wish could have lasted forever.

We returned home on the Sunday morning to pack our cases ready to drive to Portsmouth to catch our ferry to Caen. We arrived in good time and, of course, the children were desperately excited. The anticipation of spending two weeks in France was overwhelming. The ferry crossing was excellent and on arrival at Caen we set off on a long drive south through France to St Jean de Mont, on the west coast. The drive was exhausting, but we finally arrived after about six hours to find a wonderful campsite and first-class accommodation waiting for us. There was a fabulous swimming pool with several water chutes, together with a club and a games room, all of which met with the children's approval. This was without a doubt a fabulous holiday. The weather was excellent and soon we all looked very sun-kissed. During our time in France we went on various adventures around the local countryside and the beaches were fantastic.

We spent much of our time on St Jean de Mont beach. The local landscape was completely flat and the sand stretched out in either direction for miles. It was a fair walk to where the sand met the sea, but this never put the children off and we would set out our things close to the water's edge. After our previous busy weeks preparing for the wedding, there was a sense of idyllic quietness. We were holidaying out of season, so there were very few people around. Looking in any direction, there were only occasional glimpses of distant figures meandering along and the odd family engaged in similar activities to ourselves.

Stewart would play endlessly in the sand, acting out

adventures and building battle stations. I remember one day he got very panicky and upset, and when I asked him what was wrong and tried to comfort him he said, "Mummy, I've lost my Frisbee". I asked him what he had done with it. "I buried it," came the reply. I stood up straight and looked around at the sand disappearing in every direction - how were we ever going to find it again? Not surprisingly, we never did! Gemma enjoyed searching for shells and other interesting things, often using Jerzy's socks to collect them in!

All three of my children loved the water, but Jess was the water baby of the family, followed very closely by Jerzy, and they would swim for hours. No day would be complete until she'd had the chance to get wet, so every day we swam in the pool at the campsite. The water chute became a great focus for our attention, and I have to admit that even I went on it. This was not an experience that many of the other guests would forget in a hurry, as mine was the biggest tidal wave by far! At first I felt I had to accompany Stewart, who had not been confident with them in the past. That very quickly changed, however, and he soon found his confidence. I remember one particular day when he was up and down that water chute for a whole 4 ½ hours - his excitement was unending and a joy to see.

It was in this same swimming pool that Gemma, who could already swim, really developed into a strong swimmer. Her confidence grew and by the time we returned home she was capable of swimming any distance. She suddenly seemed to realise her abilities. Jess, however, was already a strong swimmer and enjoyed racing with us. She was not quite able to keep up with me, although I found it tough to stay ahead! It was early on in this holiday that Jess was to earn her nickname, a shared joke from then on. Jerzy and I were on our 'honeymoon' after all. Sometimes he would move towards me in the pool for a discreet hug or to kiss me. Always, without fail, just at that moment Jess would surface between us and laugh, peering at us cheekily from behind her goggles in the knowledge that her timing had been impeccable. Henceforth we called her 'Goggles'.

As with every family I'm sure, next on our list of priorities, behind swimming, were mealtimes. These were made up of barbecues, salads and the local cheeses, which we took great delight in hunting down. The local fresh bread was really tasty too, although I think Jerzy would tell you that the best addition to any mealtime was the local wine. We were in the heart of the Vendée region; wine was tasty, cheap and plentiful. Thus our evening meal became a bit of a ritual, the end to each perfect day. We brought a few cases home with us, too, for future enjoyment. Afterwards we would finish up in the club to enjoy the entertainment. Jess loved dressing up for the disco, as did Gemma, but Jess was becoming more grown up in her appearance and enjoyed putting on her make-up and jewellery. She made sure that she wore 'up-to-the-minute' fashionable clothes and would spend longer and longer getting ready. I think she had suddenly flourished prematurely into a teenager. The children really enjoyed the nightlife, which had a relaxed family atmosphere and added another level of enjoyment to their first experience of France. Following their late nights the children would sleep on for a short while in the mornings although Jerzy would soon have them up in order to 'hunt' for fresh croissants. There would be great disappointment if we got up too late and the rest of the campers had beaten us to it!

Within the framework of this relaxed family holiday we had several trips out to explore the area, and afterwards we often found ourselves talking and reminiscing about certain events that we had found particularly amusing. It was a trip to a wildlife park that would stick most in the minds of the children, and Jess remained traumatised by her memory of this for some time. Whilst driving through the many animal enclosures we eventually came across a paddock full of domestic animals. We were invited to get out of the car and buy some food to feed them. The problem was that there were not many visitors and I think we were the first holidaymakers the animals had seen that day. The food we bought soon had these 'friendly' goats, donkeys, ponies and sheep descending upon us from far and wide. This proved to be too much for the children, who very quickly ran in the opposite direction. Jess was set upon by a very pushy donkey, which ate the bag as well as the food and frightened her out of the field. Whenever she reminisced about this day she would call it the 'killer donkey', although she would laugh at the picture we have of it - taken from the other side of the fence!

Certainly the most picturesque location we visited was a nearby lake where we hired some pedalos and ventured quite some way from the shoreline. The scenery there was absolutely spectacular. Set in the shadows of a castle and its surrounding village, the lake curved its way through an abundance of trees which rose up dramatically on all sides. We hired two boats, one captained by Jerzy and Jess and the other by myself, Gemma and Stewart. Halfway through our adventure Gemma decided that she would like to go over to Jerzy and Jess's boat. It was so like Gemma to decide to do something without first giving it careful consideration, and no amount of persuasion could change her mind. The boats were reasonably close together, although we were in the middle of a vast expanse of water. I was half afraid to watch as Gemma leapt from one boat to the other, but in her usual style she made it safe and sound, much to my relief. Gemma was always the one to attempt the unexpected; she was never afraid of anything, possessing unusual confidence for one so young. I would sometimes cuss that free spirit of hers, but it was hard to deny that there were glimpses of me in her, a comical sense that often amused me. Jess thoroughly enjoyed the pedalos and the lake and we promised ourselves that we would go back before the end of our holiday. Unfortunately our time in France went all too quickly, however, and we were soon on our journey home without making that return visit.

Our boat home was an evening one and I remember a magical calmness: there was barely any movement at all on the surface of the sea and there were virtually no clouds in the sky, just a bright sun slowly falling. I was sat in the lounge area with Gemma and Stewart, playing a game when Jess came running to find me, with Jerzy following closely behind. She was so excited, saying "Mummy, quickly, you have to come and see." She took hold of my hand and pulled me in the direction I had to follow. She led me up an obscure staircase and out through a door. Immediately I could see why she had been so excited. I was greeted by the most amazing sunset I think I have ever seen. Jess loved nature, trees, animals, hilltops and especially sunsets. She really enjoyed seeing things of beauty stretching out before her. This sunset was completely perfect: an orange sphere enriched with glorious gold and faint wisps of cloud that caught sparkles of sunlight as it stretched across the sky. The splendour of this sight was magnified as the gentle water tentatively captured a reflection of God's painting on the sea below. The water was still so very calm, our ferry slicing through it like a knife through butter and creating only a little movement. Any noise was banished into the distance by the glory of this view and a cool breeze created only by the motion of the boat washed over our faces. I remember the joy on Jess's face, as though she had shown me something completely precious. I was aware of the beautifully tender young lady she was becoming and how honoured I felt to experience her delightful enthusiasm for this spectacular sight.

We stood for some time on this upper deck admiring this fabulous vision. Perfect is a word I have used so often, but that was how it was and how life seemed. We were all very happy: brown, having spent two glorious weeks in the sun, and content with our wonderful memories of the wedding and the holiday. It was hard to imagine that anything could ever change; we were all together, happy and healthy, with our lives before us.

Unfortunately, however, life was to change so drastically that I would reach the point when I would hardly recognise normal family life again. The wonderful times I have described would become a distant memory that was hard to cling on to, but somehow helped to keep us going as well. How wonderful that we do not know what experiences lay before us. I am so glad I was unaware that this was the calm before the storm. If I had known then that this was as good as it would get and that our time left with Jess was destined to be so short, we would not have enjoyed the spontaneity of our family life in the way that we did. With this sunset both that day and our holiday were ending, but I will always be grateful to have shared that moment with Jess.

Chapter 2

Following our wonderful holiday, Jerzy and I returned to work and the children went back to school. The spring slipped into summer. We took care of various improvements to the house, namely a conservatory, followed by copious amounts of decorating. The children continued to do well, with all three receiving nothing but the highest praise from their teachers. Stewart was finding reading difficult, although he obviously benefited from being in a small village school. The school they attended was the same village primary school I had enjoyed as a child. Nynehead had always been a focal point in my life. Although I no longer lived in the village, it was the place where I had spent my formative years and it felt wonderful to be sending my own children to the same school. Nynehead has a very close community spirit with the school at its heart and is very much an extension to the family. Jess was just finishing Year 5 and was concentrating on her SATs, which she was due to sit the following summer, 2001. All the indications were that she would do very well. She was naturally gifted in her ability, dedicated to working hard and always up for a challenge. She enjoyed school and delighted in the close friendships she built up with the children around her. Her favourite subject was art and she would delight in experimenting with colour, producing some lovely pieces of work and showing fantastic potential for the future.

The summer holiday soon arrived and long, hot days were spent enjoying the company of friends. At that time I had to work lengthy hours but fortunately my mum was able to help immensely. I had bought the house opposite my parents when my first marriage had ended; this meant that my mum was always on hand, which she enjoyed tremendously. Being a driving instructor, Jerzy was often able to arrange his lessons to fit in with whatever was going on. He would frequently take the children to the park or swimming, or arrange a surprise for me when I returned from work. I seem to remember enjoying the odd barbecue too, including wine left over from France, reminding us of our marvellous holiday. In the August Jerzy took me to Paris for a few days, which we thoroughly enjoyed. We had taken the children on honeymoon with us and therefore it was lovely to spend a few days alone together. As events were to unfold, this was the last chance that we had to delight in our own company, carefree and newly wed.

It was towards the end of August that I noticed Jess was complaining more and more of tummy pains. I took her to the doctor on several occasions, and after a brief examination I would be told that she either had a virus or the favourite suggestion seemed to be that she might be moving towards starting her periods. I had to admit that the pains did seem to come quite regularly. She would recover quickly and in between these bouts of pain she would behave like any normal ten-year-old. I therefore dismissed these earlier problems, simply giving her paracetamol regularly as suggested. The children returned to school for the autumn term and for a while there were no further difficulties. After a few weeks, when we were shopping in our local supermarket, Jess complained that her pains had returned and she needed to sit down. She asked to go and sit in the car outside, so I went with her whilst we waited for Jerzy, Gemma and Stewart to finish the shopping and go through the checkout. For several days now she had been scratching her itching legs, which at first seemed more like an irritating habit, but on the evening of our shopping trip she also started to complain of shoulder pain. I became concerned, although all these symptoms did not really make sense to me and I thought that the itching may be an allergy to washing powder or something simple like that.

I stayed home from work and arranged for Jess to see our family doctor again. He examined her but could not find anything seriously wrong, suggesting that she had strained her shoulder in some way. I accepted this because Jess was always very active and would partake in whatever opportunities came her way, so maybe she had just overdone things a little. The itching was causing Jess's scratching to break through the skin on her legs. Scabs were forming but were quickly being scratched off, the wounds were growing and her legs were often bleeding. The doctor suggested this could be due to her getting

12

too hot at night, so I changed her bedroom around to make sure she was not quite so close to the radiator. Again I tried to accept the advice given and not worry. But, as any mother knows, we care intensely about our children and sometimes you just know there is something more to it. Despite my worries, I tried to believe the simple explanations that were offered to me, but later I would come to blame myself for not questioning Jess's problems more. Again things seemed to settle down and on the whole Jess continued to be happy at school. By the weekends she would be very tired and would sleep on in the mornings, but I put this down to teenage laziness developing early.

Following the breakdown of my first marriage I encourged the children to have a lot of contact with their dad and his wider family. On Sundays he usually took the children out for the day. This was an accepted part of our routine, but Jess began not to want to go, preferring instead to rest and not really do very much. Although looking back it is easy to notice these small changes, it was not so obvious then. Jess never complained of anything specific and such a gradual change came over her that it was hard to see at first. I was to find out later that she preferred to keep her suffering to herself and, although she did not have any knowledge of her illness at this early stage, she never wanted to admit that she felt under the weather. A year or so later she did admit that she knew something was wrong but hoped it would go away. She gradually began to lose weight, unnoticed at first but eventually quite obvious. Jess had always worried that she was a little on the big side. She took after me in that department, although I never felt she had anything to worry about. When she started to get picky about the food she was eating I put this down to her wanting to lose weight. I never thought for one moment there was another underlying cause.

The changes I have described took place over the space of about six weeks, taking us to the end of October 2000, when one day I arrived home from work to find Jess waiting on the doorstep for me. She was crying and desperate for a hug. In her distress she tried to tell me what had happened, but she was afraid and very muddled. I guided her inside to find my mum, hoping to get to understand what was going on. Mum soon put me in the picture and explained that Jess had become upset at

13

school and was experiencing pain. She had spoken to one of the teachers, who had noticed that her eyes had turned yellow. My mother had picked the children up from school and had taken Jess straight to the doctor. He had examined her and felt she may be suffering from hepatitis A, which is apparently very common. She had a faint yellow glow about her and I could see that the whites of her eyes were indeed slightly yellow. An appointment had been made for her to attend the nurse's clinic for a blood test, which the doctor felt would confirm the problem. He had reassured my mum it was not serious but it might take her some time to get over. As hepatitis A is fairly contagious, I notified the school in the morning and decided to keep Gemma and Stewart at home just in case they had it as well. Jess needed lots of reassurance and love. She became very down and would sleep for long spells during the day. I found it hard to work and was grateful for the support of my employer, who allowed me time off to be with Jess. I sat with her for hours just holding her and being there for her. I was upset to see her this way, but allowed myself to be reassured that although she would feel ill for some time she would get better eventually, helped along with some tender loving care.

Jess had the blood test and we eagerly awaited the result. I spent a lot of time reassuring her, reiterating what the doctor had said: "It is remarkably common but it might take some time for you to feel better." We talked about how she would need quite a long time off school as she would feel very tired. She was worried about getting behind with her SATs, as she had set herself very high targets. Gemma and Stewart returned to school as they had shown no signs of yellow colouring and seemed perfectly well. However, by the time I received a phone call from the doctor with Jess's blood results, she had deteriorated still further. She was now extremely yellow and the scratched areas on her legs were getting worse. Her itching had spread to other parts of her body and she was constantly digging at her wounds even in her sleep. Consequently, she rarely seemed to rest and I encouraged her to wear mittens in bed in an attempt to protect her wounded skin. Her eyes had long since lost their sparkle, her lids consistently weighing heavy with sleep and progressively she lost her appetite becoming boney and gaunt.

The results were a bit of a shock: they had not shown that Jess had hepatitis but that her liver function was all over the place. What did this mean? I started to panic at this point - if she didn't have hepatitis then what was wrong? The doctor reassured me that he had been advised Jess should have another blood test and therefore another appointment was made. And so we would have to wait another week for more results. I started to feel as though somewhere a clock was ticking and time was running out.

Jess slept for such long periods in the day and I was at home, so I took to decorating her bedroom. This way I could keep a close eye on her but it also gave me something to do. I was out of my mind with worry by this point. It seemed strange with her sleeping in the middle of the room and me painting around her, and I remember thinking: what if the doctor is wrong; what if she is dying; how would I know? I know now that I should have made more of a fuss. I should have realised there was something more and I will never forgive myself for allowing further reassurance to be enough.

As Jess slept I watched her yellow collouring gradually intensify and her arms were rarely still as she continued to wrestle with her persistent itching. She had gouged great wounds on her legs, feet, toes and arms that were constantly bleeding or oozing yellow stuff. Even wearing shoes on her feet had become painful. By now she was sleeping her days away and hardly eating or drinking anything. It was clear that she was suffering. I felt completely helpless - just what was I supposed to do? Should I listen to the reassurances or follow my instincts and make more of a fuss? Whilst waiting for the second lot of blood test results I phoned our out-of-hours doctors' service and asked if she could be seen at the hospital. After explaining our situation I was told, "There is little point in bringing her to me. I will only be looking at a yellow child!" I remember feeling quite shocked and unsupported in that moment, anger still sits in my heart when I reflect on those words in disbelief that anyone could have been that harsh. The next day I spoke to our doctor again, who tried to reiterate that her symptoms were a side effect of the jaundice and in time she would begin to feel better. I was growing tired of his reassurances now and all he could suggest for the itching was Calamine lotion.

I sat with Jess constantly whilst she slept, and I could not lose the thought that there was more than I knew. I had experienced a distressing dream several months earlier that had had a huge effect on me. However, in time I had dismissed it as being completely irrelevant. Suddenly I remembered this dream and it filled me with fear. Looking back, I think it was recalling this that woke me up to myself and suddenly inspired me to start listening to my own judgement. I had dreamed that I saw Jess lying lifeless in a white coffin, her skin pale like porcelain, but there had been no explanation of what had happened. Why had this vision suddenly come back to haunt me now?

It was now two weeks before Christmas Day 2000, as I was helping Jess into bed, she complained of intense pain. She said it went all the way around to her back. She told me that she was afraid of the pain, and did not want to go to bed and be separated from me. Her face echoed that pain as though she were being tortured. I had reached my limit; I could not simply watch and do nothing anymore. Perhaps I had waited too long already and enough was enough. I wrapped her in a blanket and carried her frail, weakened body to the car. It was very late into the night, but I drove her to the hospital where I insisted that she saw a doctor straight away. I made it quite clear that I was not leaving until someone did something for her. I think Jess found my behaviour quite amusing: "Wow, Mum!" was the expression she used. I remember smiling quietly back at her, but in all seriousness her condition was now extremely worrying. She had not eaten or drunk anything that day and she looked terrible. I blamed myself for allowing this to go on too long. The doctor that saw her was a kindly gentleman who took great care while examining her and immediately decided to admit her for further investigation. He felt that the original diagnosis was probably correct, but at least we would get Jess's blood results back more quickly and ultimately receive confirmation of the diagnosis. And so we made our way to the children's ward. This was the first time she had been in hospital and I think she was a little amazed by all the attention. She remarked several times how she couldn't wait to tell her friends

16

that she had spent the night in hospital!

By now it was about 11.00 p.m., the main lights were out and all her initial investigations were done with the illumination of a bedside lamp. It was not until the following morning that we would start to get to know the nurses and staff on the ward, and these late few hours were a blur of mixed emotions and examinations. I gradually became more worried when the doctors obviously noticed something about the feel of her tummy. When they tapped it with a finger the tone changed, which again I noticed. After what seemed like hours Jess fell asleep in my arms, comforted by painkillers and some anti-itch medicine called Piriton. A drip had been put up to ensure that her fluids were restored to an acceptable level. It was clear that she was more comfortable now; her body no longer seemed rigid with pain as she had relaxed into sleep. I had told her I would have to go home as we had brought nothing with us, and I promised I would return before she woke up in the morning. I was feeling really lost and alone in coping with the possibilities, scared to imagine what might be wrong. However, Jess seemed content for the moment and certainly peaceful, so I quietly collected my coat.

As I was leaving, I was met by the doctor. She explained to me that there are two types of jaundice: one caused by an illness like hepatitis, and the other caused by an obstruction. Jess's jaundice was presenting as the obstructive type, which meant there was something blocking her bile duct. I understood instantly what she was trying so kindly and gently to say, even though she never said it out loud. From then on I realised they thought Jess had a tumour. An appointment had been made for an ultrasound examination the following day (Sunday). I walked off down the corridor, tears streaming down my face, her words repeating over and over in my head. All the unthinkable 'what ifs?' and 'whys?' taking over my whole thought process. Why had I not brought her sooner? Why had it taken me so long to realise that something serious was wrong? Why? I loved Jess so much; she was everything to me.

I felt so very tired; a muddle of thoughts and nothing made sense at all. Suddenly I stopped walking and looked up, realising that I had no idea where I was and there was no one

17

around. I had been so taken up with my emotions that I had just kept walking, totally oblivious as to my direction. I turned round and walked back, trying to retrace my steps. Eventually I found where I had gone wrong and discovered my car totally alone in the car park and waiting patiently for my return. My oblivious state seemed to continue and how I drove home that night I have no idea. I got to bed at about 2.00 a.m. and was up again at around 6.00 a.m. I don't know if I slept at all that night, plagued as I was by words and thoughts running away with themselves. I tried to be objective and tell myself that I must wait and see what the scan showed.

Jerzy agreed to stay and take care of Gemma and Stewart so that I could return to the hospital. Remembering my promise to Jess, I was determined to be there before she woke up. I left promptly without having any breakfast, as I was eager not to be late. I walked quietly onto the ward and I remember feeling relieved that Jess was still sleeping peacefully. I pulled up a big, comfortable chair and relaxed into it, waiting for her to stir. As I watched her sleeping my eyes filled with tears, but I tried hard not to cry; I wanted to stay positive for Jess. I was thankful that she seemed so peaceful. She was no longer fidgeting to scratch her wounds and she seemed genuinely relaxed and deeply asleep. I reflected on our relationship - how we laughed together and enjoyed the same things. Her artistic abilities mirrored my own and we shared many happy times being creative together. I was desperately tired but too troubled with my thoughts to try to doze in the chair. Every time I checked the clock only minutes had passed and yet my mind was racing. Soon Jerzy crept in to join me. It was then that Jess finally woke up, extremely pleased to see us both and anxious to talk about her experiences of hospital life to Jerzy.

Through the course of the morning we met various members of staff, who took great delight in distracting Jess from her problems. Jackie, our nurse for that shift, soon introduced herself and became a friend to Jess, and she would remain a good friend to us both throughout Jess's illness. Jackie's strength and dedication were truly remarkable and Jess took to her instantly. She was kept busy with various 'arty' things to do and delighted in any suggested activities. Ann, another kindly nurse, would appear from time to time to remind Jess that she needed to try to drink. This became a bit of a game to Jess and she laughed at Ann's persistent badgering. Ann, too, would become a predominant figure in Jess's care. She often tried to offer me support and she seemed to know without my having to say anything just how hard it all was for me.

Jessica's scan had been arranged for midday and by this time we had been joined by the children's father. Dr Pullaperuma, the consultant we had met during the night, also 'happened to be passing' at the same time and joined us in the scanning room. The scan lasted a good while. As it was a Sunday the department was deserted apart from us, which felt a bit strange. It was clear that they had discovered something, because the doctor conducting the scan and Dr Pullaperuma seemed to have a lot to chat about. Jess found the procedure uncomfortable and was glad when they had finished. Nothing much was said and we returned to the ward. Later Dr Pullaperuma came and found us and took us to one side. He explained they could see that Jess's liver was not normal; it was enlarged and hard. They couldn't tell us any more than that, but arranged for her to have a CT scan on the Monday morning when hopefully they would be able to make a clearer diagnosis. We were obviously very worried, but Dr Pullaperuma was reassuring and tried to give us this news in a sensitive way. I think I had already worked out the rest and certainly, judging by the looks on their faces, the staff already knew what was wrong but nobody wanted to be the first to say anything. We spent another agonising night in anticipation of her scan, but Jess was completely unaware of our worries. She was enjoying herself with wonderful members of the nursing team who had seemingly taken her under their wing.

The next day Jerzy and I accompanied Jess to the X-ray department where she would have her CT scan. She was nervous about it; everything was new to her at this stage. Little did she know then that lying in a scanner would become something of a regular occurrence. She lay perfectly still and I held on to her feet for moral support. The scans seemed to take ages and again Jess became uncomfortable due to lying for a long time on a flat, hard surface. The man that had confidently helped to set Jess up on the scanner returned after a while to announce that we were all done. He had joked a little previously but was now unable to look me in the eye or even raise his gaze from the floor. I was instinctively aware the news was not good. Dr Pullaperuma also magically appeared, saying that he 'just happened to be passing'. He announced he wanted to see Jerzy and I after lunch. We went to the hospital café together, but it felt really strange. Jerzy and I were afraid to talk about our fears and were trying to be chatty with Jess, who was still blissfully unaware of our concerns. I knew I wanted to be honest, but I didn't want to speculate and cause unnecessary distress.

Our meeting came all too soon and we were shown Jess's scan pictures. Our worst nightmares were sadly realised. Dr Pullaperuma confirmed that she had an enormous tumour, taking up virtually all of her liver and about 18 centimetres in diameter. We both became tearful at the confirmation of this news, although it was really not that much of a surprise by then but more a realisation of the truth. I tried to jump ahead and asked if she was going to be all right. Dr Pullaperuma preferred to stick to the facts and reiterated what they knew, confirming that she would have to be transferred to Bristol Children's Hospital for a biopsy in order to confirm the diagnosis. Beyond that he was not prepared in his professional capacity to speculate. He was a lovely man with such a kind face, and he remained in contact throughout Jess's story and showed genuine compassion for her dilemma. We would have to wait for confirmation that a bed would be available for her the next day (Tuesday). Jess was then brought in to join us and she was shown the scan pictures. Dr Pullaperuma discussed it with her, referring to the tumour as 'a lump', which somehow did not sound as bad. Jess took it all in and didn't really react. I believe her calmness came from genuinely not knowing anything about cancer. This lump had no sinister connotations at all and she took everything in her stride.

We returned to the parents' lounge so that we could be left on our own for a moment. I talked to Jess about what had been said. Christmas was just a little less than two weeks away and this was her greatest fear - she wanted to be home for Christmas. We cried together and I held her close, but I knew my tears were for a different reason. She cried for Christmas, because she would miss her home and her friends; I cried because I feared for her life - I wanted to protect her and I couldn't bear the thought of losing her. Very soon we were joined by a number of relatives who had come to visit Jess, not realising that their timing was more than awkward. We announced what had happened and everyone was taken over by a mixture of disbelief and immense sadness. I quickly rescued Jess and took her back to her hospital bed where she found a bouquet of flowers waiting. These had been sent by my cousin, Andrew, and she was so pleased to receive them: "It's the first time anyone has ever sent me flowers!" she joked. My cousin had not been aware of our news but his floral gesture was so timely.

It seemed no time at all before Sarah arrived. Jerzy had called her. She gave me a very welcome hug and I remember feeling so relieved that she was there. Jess seemed to be feeling much stronger now and she was enjoying the distraction of being able to play with the girls. They were such lovely friends and I think she really appreciated their visiting her. They picked up her spirits as only children know how. Sarah and I walked off for a while to talk; we cried a little too. I spoke to her about my suspicion that Jess had cancer. It was the first time I had spoken that dreaded 'c' word out loud. Certainly there was no doubt that she was seriously ill. We spoke about how hard it would be for Jess, so far from home, friends and family, particularly with Christmas such a short time away. I knew it would be difficult for both of us but Dr Pullaperuma had been clear; we had no choice. Thank goodness for friends like Sarah, she was so very supportive and promised to help look after Gemma and Stewart while I was away; she knew it broke my heart to leave them.

Jess fell asleep early, exhausted by the events of the day as she had not rested at all. She was full of anticipation about Bristol Children's Hospital but was too tired to be unduly worried. Final confirmation of the availability of a bed would come in the morning and we had elected to drive her straight there rather than go by ambulance.

When everyone had gone and Jess was asleep, I was once again left alone with my thoughts. Exhausted, I slumped into the chair next to her bed. I had promised her I would not leave her alone that night. Silently I had promised in my heart that I would never leave her; no matter what it took I was determined to remain by her side. I watched her sleeping and traced every line of her beautiful face. How could life change so much in just a few days? Ann caught up with me again as I made my way along the corridor to get a cup of tea. It was very late and the ward was quiet and virtually in darkness. She asked if I was all right and I told her how exhausted and worried I felt. I was obviously tearful, which was hardly surprising really as quality sleep was a distant memory. Then I said what I felt everyone had been avoiding saying: "I think Jess has got cancer". Ann never said yes, but neither did she say no. What she did do was reassure me that if Jess needed chemotherapy she would be able to return to Taunton for treatment. I took this to mean that my conclusion was probably right. Then she said something that I often reflected on and that turned out to be very true: "You'll surprise yourself and will find strength in places you never knew existed." Right now I didn't feel very strong, but I knew I had to be so for Jess. I didn't know what was ahead, but I knew I had to do my best. Ann gave me a big hug - she obviously thought I needed it and she was probably right. I had yet another sleepless night ahead of me: my thoughts and fears for Jess were still paramount in my mind, a jumble of the day's events and unspoken words. I wondered if I was going to Bristol with Jess to watch her die. Would she ever come home? At that time I thought I would never sleep well again.

Chapter 3

Tuesday morning felt very strange as we waited for the announcement that a bed was available at Bristol for Jess. We were sad to be leaving an environment in which we felt comfortable, but we knew that Jess had to go to Bristol for us to stand a hope of her ever getting better.

I had spent the night in Musgrove with Jess, much of it by her bedside. I had cried quietly to myself, but I tried not to show my fear in front of Jess. Once she was awake and dressed I packed our things in anticipation of our move. She played happily with the play therapists and seemed oblivious to her problems, and for the moment that seemed to be for the best. Although she was a clever girl, I did not want to burden her with our unsubstantiated fears. Jerzy and I had discussed what we should say to her and we had agreed we would remain as cheerful as possible around her. Until we had received a firm diagnosis we could not elaborate on what she already knew.

Whilst Jess remained playing happily on the ward I returned home briefly to pack some things for both Jess and myself. I decided to pack quite a lot of clothes, as I had no idea what the facilities would be like and when I might next encounter a washing machine. I packed plenty of pyjamas for Jess and, as it was now so close to Christmas, I found some fairy lights and some tinsel and packed those as well. I wanted to decorate her bed once we were settled on the ward, as I was determined she would still enjoy Christmas. It was at this point that I sat Gemma and Stewart down and explained as clearly as possible what had happened to Jess. I explained that Jess was very ill indeed and that she had a 'lump' in her tummy. I told them we had to go to another hospital in Bristol for the doctors to make Jess better. Gemma was seven and Stewart was six years old at this time, so their comprehension of the events was limited, but we cried together and I cuddled them both and told them how much I loved them. I told them that I would speak to them as often as I could on the telephone and that Jerzy would bring them up to see us both. They didn't want me to go; Stewart was almost

23

hysterical and it was extremely difficult to leave, but I was aware that Jerzy and Andrew would be waiting for me to return.

What a dreadful thing for a mother to have to do. To leave Gemma and Stewart behind tore my heart out, but my instinct was to be with Jess, so I had no choice. I gathered my things and walked to the car. I was torn in two. I hated having to leave and Stewart was clinging on to me crying, "Don't go, Mummy; I don't want you to go." I hugged him goodbye and my mum tried to pacify him for me, and eventually I was able to begin my journey back to the children's ward. I felt traumatised by this separation - poor Stewie was little more than a baby really and he didn't understand. Before I left, my mum asked if there was anything she could do to help. "Please watch out for Gemma and Stewart and take care of them for me, as I don't know how long we will be gone," had been my answer. I drove off down the road, crying again; my sadness at leaving my two youngest children a physical pain that I could hardly bear. I had spent so much time in tears over the previous few days and my final words to my mother echoed in my head: "I don't know how long we will be gone." On my drive back to the hospital I came to the conclusion that Jess and I could be in Bristol for a long time and crying all the time was not going to help matters. Apart from a few occasions when I attempted to comfort her and we openly shared our tears, on the whole I had prevented myself from crying in front of Jess. I had always been known for my strength of character and determination, and now was the time I would have to use these qualities to their extreme. Jess needed to lean on me and I wasn't going to let her down. By the time I found myself walking up the corridor towards the children's ward I had put my distress at leaving the children to one side for the moment and I was ready to fight this. No matter what it took, I would be there for my darling Jess and I would do whatever was needed to help her, although at this stage a definitive diagnosis was the next step.

We took Jess to the car in a wheelchair as she was now too feeble to walk any distance. I remembered how only a few months previously she had moaned about being overweight; now she appeared bony and yellow, a mere shadow of her former healthy and vibrant self.

It was pouring with rain as we set off up the motorway towards Bristol Children's Hospital. Andrew followed behind in his car. The rain so aptly summed up our mood. We all tried to stay bright and cheery for Jess, but inwardly we cried almost as relentlessly as the rain. I sat alongside Jess and she cuddled up to me for support. The cannula that had been used for copious blood tests had been in Jess's arm for several days now and had been left in place for her treatment at Bristol, so she focused her anger on the discomfort it gave her. Jess had been almost proud of it initially, but now she was fed up and miserable and would have done anything for someone to remove it for her.

After our seemingly endless journey through that dreadful weather, we arrived outside the Children's Hospital. As it was positioned awkwardly on a very steep hill with limited parking facilities, Jerzy decided to drop Jess and myself directly outside and then try to find somewhere to leave the car. We made our way as quickly as we could to the main entrance, and Jess was clearly glad to rest a while once we were inside. A kindly receptionist found a wheelchair for her and called for someone from Ward 31 to come and find us. By the time a nurse had arrived, Jerzy and Andrew had caught up.

There was a huge difference between Bristol Children's Hospital and our own Children's Unit at Taunton's Musgrove Park Hospital. The harsh reality of this run down old victorian building was a huge shock to me, but I quickly learnt that a new Children's Hospital was nearing completion at the bottom of the hill. The state of the present building was dreadful; if I hadn't witnessed it myself I would never have believed it. All the funding was clearly being directed towards the new building and the staff and patients in the old hospital were having to 'make do' in the meantime.

When we left the lift on the top floor, we found the corridor to be lined with old beds, cots, unused furniture and equipment. There were a few wheelchairs parked directly outside the ward of which, I discovered later, only one worked effectively as either the tyres were flat or bits were missing. The corridor was filthy, the floor was disgusting and this general state of uncleanliness continued onto the ward: there was clutter everywhere and space was obviously a big issue. My first impressions were of complete horror. All the beds were occupied by desperately ill children and surounded by piles of posessions including rolled up bedding, toys and spare clothes. Concerned famillies were trying to make the best of their limited allocated spaces, many had clearly been residents there for some while. The sadness of this sight overwhelmed me, being reminiscent of a refugee camp. However, this first impression of the hospital was to be proved unfounded. Yes, the conditions that had to be tolerated by both patients and staff alike were truly awful, but Jess was to receive care that was second to none. Both the nursing staff and the consultants were so very dedicated and cared intensely for the children that sadly found themselves in need of treatment on this oncology ward. I learned so much from the other families, too, as I made friends with other mothers, and in many respects the only way to survive this time was to join together - a special kindness and complete understanding that bound us all. We all felt each other's pain and tried to help where we could. We comforted one another and occasionally we even laughed together.

Jess was shown to a bed right next to the busy nursing station and various nurses and doctors came to make our acquaintance. They confirmed the fact that Jess had a tumour in her liver and a slot was found for theatre the next day. Jess was going to have an open liver biopsy, which would enable a diagnosis to be made. I got Jess unpacked and settled in whilst she watched her own personal television. This was one thing that Jess rejoiced in - her own personal television and video, which she had not had on the ward in Taunton.

From what I could make out, there were two oncology wards at this Children's Hospital and ward 31 catered for the younger age group. She appeared to be almost the oldest on the ward. Opposite us was a dear little baby called Sophie, who had such a sunny disposition that she stole everybody's hearts. Her mother, Nicola, and I quickly became good friends. All the children on the ward and those that were isolated in side rooms were in various stages of hair loss and were clearly showing those very sad symptoms that we associate with cancer and leukaemia. You would have thought it was a sad place, and initially it was a very sad place to me. But as relationships developed and I watched the staff at work, it wasn't a sad place at all: everyone was full of hope for the future. Not one of those children was giving up; everyone was taking their own illness step by step, supported by the close bond of their own family.

Jerzy, Andrew and I stayed with Jess initially, although because poor Jess was trying to come to terms with all that was happening I persuaded Jerzy and Andrew to give us both some space so that we could talk quietly together. The last few days had been such a blur and I was frightened that Jess had initially retreated into a shell, and understandably so, as even I had found our arrival on this ward daunting and poor Jess had not said much at all. Jerzy went to find us some sandwiches for tea and Andrew went to try to find some accommodation for himself. I talked to Jess quietly on my own. I thought she might have been worried about the children she could see around her and maybe realised more clearly her own situation. From our conversation it was clear Jess had no comprehension of what 'oncology' meant, a word we had heard a lot over those few days. She did not ask, so I did not say. She was more concerned about being away from Gemma and Stewart and missing school (she wanted so badly to do well in her SATs), and one of the nurses had said we would be there a couple of weeks at least, which meant she would be in hospital over Christmas.

Christmas, as with most families, was our favourite time of year and I always tried to make each Christmas better than the one before. Financially we had found life easier since Jerzy had been with us and so we hoped that this Christmas, our first since the wedding, would be special. Therefore Jess was really looking forward to the festivities and the thought of being stuck in this ward, which at this stage felt very uninviting, was not to her liking at all. We talked at length about it and I tried to make her realise that, no matter what, we would all be together and if she could not go home for Christmas then we would bring Christmas to her. The thought of Jerzy dressed up as Santa put a smile back on her face and I managed to reassure her that Christmas would still be special. She was anxious about her operation as well, as she had never had an anaesthetic before, and I tried to allay her fears.

Very soon we met Jessica's surgeon for the biopsy, Mr Spicer, who would become a prominent figure in her treatment and was a real character. Every time he came to the ward he wore a different tie, some of which would flash or play music, and Jess found this an endearing quality in a grown-up. She quickly learned to trust him as he explained the procedure for the operation the next day. Mr Spicer seemed a tremendously sincere man. He spoke to Jess in a calm and straightforward manner and she asked lots of questions about the operation. She was a clever child and he quickly realised that this was the case and seemed to sum up her personality instantly. When he spoke to me he explained some of the risks, including that of bleeding, and how difficult it was to operate on the liver. I signed the consent form, knowing that the biopsy would be the only way to diagnose this tumour properly, although I was inwardly terrified of signing my precious child over for the first time. Mr Spicer seemed to know how difficult it was for me and gave me a knowing glance that said so much without actually speaking the words in front of Jess.

Jessica had picked up on the word 'risk' through listening to our conversation and it was not until a later stage that I would realise how much this one word had affected her. We managed to find a couple of camp bed mattresses and Jerzy and I slept on the floor next to Jess's bed. There was a lack of bedding for parents and I never managed to lay claim to a pillow in the whole time we spent on that ward. We found a couple of blankets and I folded up a soft fleece to use as a pillow. If Jess wanted anything she would lean over the side of the bed and poke me. This became a bit of a standing joke, but she wanted me near so I didn't mind.

Other parents slept either under or next to their child's bed. One lady had a particularly small area and her baby was in a cot. Because she was so small herself she actually slept in the cot with her child! Her husband slept underneath with his feet sticking out across the corridor. Nobody seemed to mind where you decided to sleep; the important thing was to get comfortable with the small amount of bedding that was available and make the most of it. I find it amazing just where you can sleep when tiredness takes over. I found that I developed the skill of being able to switch off to all the noises around me apart from Jess and

I would sleep because my body needed to rest. This was not relaxed sleep, as I could be up and on my feet at a moment's notice if necessary, it was just a state of mind that allowed my body to rest although my soul was still active.

In the morning I was up and in the shower before Jess woke up. The one parent shower for the whole building was situated on the floor below and I learned that if you got up early enough you were sure to get there before anyone else. After about 7.30 a.m. it was constantly occupied and various queues would form outside. The downfall of being first in the shower was that the hot water had not found its way along the old pipes, so the water remained cold for a good while. However, I always came out feeling refreshed and, as the ward was so warm, the cold shower served to revive me a little for the day ahead.

This Wednesday morning I then got Jess ready for surgery, helping her to bathe and put on her gown. This was a similar gown to those worn by adults in that it did not fasten at the back, although the material was more suited to a child. However, the design was still awkward and, as Jess put it, "not very private"! Jess was not best pleased about this, but if she took hold of the back and pulled it around her she did not have a problem. The bathroom was completely full of clutter, so much so that we could only access one side of the bath. It was full of redundant equipment and high chairs, but if you looked past all that the walls were decorated with teddy bears. In fact, someone had painted teddy bears all over the ward and continued the theme into the bathroom - what dedication by someone to decide to brighten up the ward in this way, as they were definitely hand-painted, not the stickers that can so easily be bought these days.

Jess waited for what seemed like ages for someone to come and take her to theatre. We met one of the first hospital teachers Jess would get to know. She was a lovely lady, who quickly realised that Jess needed something to take her mind off her forthcoming operation. Jess had not been allowed anything to eat or drink and was feeling very sad about this. To cheer her up, a laptop computer appeared and was plugged into a socket on the wall. Jess was thrilled with this and she worked intently through a programme that dealt with wild animals and their habitat. It was just what she needed, and I was so grateful.

29

The time passed much more quickly now and soon a porter arrived to take Jess to theatre. I accompanied her, leaving Andrew and Jerzy on the ward. We were met by an anaesthetist in the theatre's reception area. Through the partially open doors I could hear students talking somewhat bluntly about Jess's biopsy, so I kept talking to Jess to take her ears away from it. I told her how much I loved her, how brave she was and that I would be there when she woke up. As the anaesthetist injected a syringe filled with a white substance Jess almost immediately fell asleep. Tears rolled down my face as I said, "Please take good care of her for me." I stood in the corridor outside the theatre and cried to myself. I had never been in the situation of having to hand Jess's life over in such a way before and I felt so helpless. The nurse who had accompanied me offered reassurance and steered me back to the ward for a cup of tea. She explained that once Jess was back in recovery someone would either phone up or come and get me, so that I could be there for her when she woke up.

Her operation took about an hour, not long really, but it was the longest hour I have ever spent. Jerzy and I sat by Jess's empty bed and spoke to neighbouring parents. I could not leave the ward; I needed to be close at hand. Andrew went out for a walk, as I think he found it hard to sit still. It was hard for him suddenly to be thrown back into the situation of spending so much time with me again and in such unspeakably awful circumstances. I also found it hard, but I was always aware that Jess was his daughter too and if he wanted to be there then he should be there. Jess loved Jerzy and Andrew and therefore it was important for all three of us to stand together to support her, no matter how difficult it was to achieve. Every minute of my separation from Jess seemed like an eternity and I was almost beside myself with worry when a call finally came. I was escorted to recovery and immediately found Jess without further direction.

They had made a large vertical incision in the middle of her abdomen, and she was in a lot of pain. I held her hand and spoke gently to her in an attempt to calm her down. Little I did made any difference to her and the nursing team quickly realised that she would need some additional pain management. Organising the morphine driver seemed to take forever and, by the time we were almost ready to go back to the ward, word came that Andrew and Jerzy were very worried. When I checked the clock almost an hour and a half had gone by since my arrival in recovery. Finally Jess was calm and comfortable enough to return to the ward, although moving her to her bed from the trolley proved a painful experience.

Once in bed she slept peacefully, her intense yellow colouring was now strikingly obvious against the starched white sheets of her bed. I never left her side and I would spend hours knelt on the floor with one arm around her and the other holding her hand. She would stir intermittently for a sip of water and to check I was still there. It was so sad to see her this way. Jerzy had to leave to go home, as he had some driving lessons the next day and he needed to be there for Gemma and Stewart as well. Andrew had decided he would stay until Saturday, and he had managed to find a bed and breakfast just up the road from the hospital. I wanted to stay on the ward and, in many ways, I gained strength from talking to the other families. The results of the biopsy would not be known for a couple of days, so I focused my attention on taking care of Jess. The operation had really taken it out of her and she slept almost continuously for about three days, and following that she would be awake for only short spells.

I learned about a wonderful place, CLIC House, run by a charity called CLIC (Cancer and Leukaemia in Children). Most of the families on the ward had been allocated a room there and the accommodation was supposed to be like that of a hotel, with somewhere to cook meals and enjoy a nice bath or shower, and also washing and drying facilities. If Jessica's diagnosis was one of cancer then we would be allocated a room at CLIC House. I dreaded the thought that this would be the diagnosis, but Nicola obviously enjoyed her trip there every day for a shower and a rest whilst her husband took over taking care of Sophie. The social worker came to visit me and confirmed that I would only be allocated a room once Jessica's diagnosis was confirmed. She was a helpful lady and set about filling in forms for financial support and help of all kinds.

On the Friday (two days after surgery) Jessica was still sleepy.

She was again scratching her itchy wounds incessantly and by now some of them were full-thickness open wounds that oozed and bled onto the sheets. The jaundice was still persisting and obviously caused her a great amount of discomfort, and it was this that was adding to her sleepiness. Whilst I was attending to her, Mr Spicer appeared and announced that he had some news from her biopsy. We arranged for him to return at about 5.00 p.m. to discuss everything with both Andrew and myself. I dreaded this meeting, but by the same token we needed to know the results. I was very aware that up to now nothing had been done to try to treat Jess in any way. So I focused on waiting for 5.00 p.m. to arrive.

However, at about 3.30 p.m. the social worker reappeared and handed me an envelope, saying, "I was so sorry to hear your news." I looked at her blankly and she continued, "Here are your keys". I was still speechless. "Here are your keys to CLIC House." I was completely stunned, overwhelmed by intense fear and sadness: she had not only handed me some keys, by doing so she had told me my daughter had cancer.

The conversation that followed was muddled. She realised that I had not yet been told the diagnosis and then tried to say that the keys were being given to me because we were a long way from home. I knew this to be a lie because everyone had told me how strictly access to the house was regulated. This was a really unfortunate miss in communication which was no ones fault but a truely distressing experience for me. Jess was still asleep. The social worker left. I quietly fell into a sea of silent tears.

When 5.00 p.m. came, nothing that followed was really a surprise anymore. I felt so numb from the events of the afternoon that I was already prepared for the answers I had waited so long to hear. Andrew was there and we followed Mr Spicer into a nearby office. Another consultant was there too, who was standing in for the lady that would oversee Jess's care when she returned from holiday, and a nurse was also present. Mr Spicer sensitively announced that Jess's tumour was malignant - the news that I had so dreaded. It was apparently very large and essentially unlike anything he had seen before. It had not been possible to reveal the complete story with the biopsy and therefore samples had been sent off to various places all around the world for further analysis. Tears ran down my face as this final confirmation came, but I was not beyond speaking and I almost spitefully said, "I don't care about any of that. I just want to know if my daughter is going to die." The lady consultant answered this calmly, realising how desperate we both felt - who wouldn't? "We need to wait for further information from the biopsy results and then we will talk to you about this. At the moment we don't have enough knowledge." One positive note was that the samples taken from one side of the liver were normal, which meant that surgery might be possible at some time. Mr Spicer was in contact with a further surgeon in Birmingham, as he would not be able to operate on Jess himself - the surgery would be too risky. We needed to wait to hear what this surgeon, Mr de Ville de Goyet, would say.

Mr Spicer felt that Jess should be told. I agreed that she should know, but I felt she needed to recover from her surgery and I wanted to talk to her quietly about it; I wanted to tell her myself. It was agreed to leave it for now. I choked back my tears and tried to appear bright for Jess, who was still so very sleepy. She wanted to know why I had been crying, in response I tried to make light of my tearfulness but I know she saw right through me. Mr Spicer also came to see Jess but not before he disappeared for a short while. I think he had found the news hard to break to us and he needed to regain his composure.

And so it was confirmed that my darling Jessica had liver cancer. It is so hard to explain what that felt like. On the one hand, I was relieved that at least I knew what we were dealing with. Talking to the other residents on the ward had served to give me encouragement and strength. On the other hand, I was in shock that in the space of seemingly only a few days my world had changed beyond recognition. My daughter was seriously ill and I had to find the strength both to talk to her about it and to fight it with her. My children were my whole life and the possibility of losing Jess was too much for me to digest. I needed to gather a sense of myself again, to find my own strength in order to encourage strength and hope in Jess. I decided to give her the chance to recover from her operation and then I would talk to her about it all. Mr Spicer had felt that Jess was old enough to be involved in her treatment and to understand what was happening to her, and I agreed totally. It was not really a question of whether she should know more, but rather a question of choosing the right moment to tell her.

Chapter 4

Over that weekend Jess recovered a little more each day and became more wakeful. She was still yellow and very thin, but the pain she had suffered following surgery had subsided. She was able to play with the other children on the ward and enjoyed joining in with various organised activities. We talked a lot and she always wanted me close for reassurance. Her consultant returned from holiday and reiterated how difficult it was to make a detailed diagnosis. Based on the information that they had already received, Jess's tumour was extremely rare, but they wanted to wait a little longer for more advice to come through.

She was a very professional lady, confident in her advice and obviously very knowledgeable. Although at this stage just another doctor, later she would become very prominent in Jess's care. I had seen so many people and listened to many doctors confirming this and that, and it seemed she was just another to bring me sad news. She did say they were very aware they had not done anything as yet towards treating Jess's illness. So far they had only tried to control Jess's pain and therefore the proposed plan was to start her on some chemotherapy by Thursday. It was already Monday of that week, so she wanted me to tell Jess what was happening and explain to her about the side effects of the medicines they hoped to use. She offered to do this for me, but I wanted Jess to be able to trust me and I needed to explain why I had not told her until now. She had to know everything so that we could work through this together.

In the short time we had been in Bristol Children's Hospital, Jess had not openly compared herself to the other children on the ward, although she would find out what was wrong with the children she played with - she knew that Sophie had leukaemia, for instance. Jess had identified the chemotherapy and the way it was administered through drips, and had remarked on the amazing colours of the medicines that were used. However, never did she ask me if she had cancer, although her consultants felt she possibly had questions she had not been brave enough to ask. I took time out to think and walked along the road to find CLIC House. Although I had been given the key on the Friday and it was now the following Monday afternoon, I had only just found the confidence to leave Jess for the first time. She seemed happy with her new-found friends and I needed time to get it clear in my mind how I was going to talk to Jess.

It was still raining; it had seemed to rain forever. There was a chilly bite to the air, so I walked briskly to try to keep warm. The cold almost served to wake me up; if I felt cold I wasn't dreaming. Words kept flying around my head: how was I going to talk to Jess? I had never had a problem speaking to her about things before, yet for the first time in my life words failed me. I arrived at CLIC House and pulled the key from my pocket, my fingers were numb with the cold and my hair was so wet that water dripped onto my face. The big, heavy door opened easily, and as the gap widened a gush of warm air flooded out to greet me. I walked into the hallway and pushed open the door immediately in front of me. I had found the living room, which was large and beautifully furnished. Toys were positioned tidily around the room: huge cuddly animals, garages, cars, dolls and all manner of games; there was even a pool table and a Subbuteo football game. Dominating one corner of this inviting family room was an enormous Christmas tree. It was covered in shimmering lights and fabulous decorations - so brilliant a sight that it held my gaze. There were no other lights on, the house was completely silent and the room was filled with absolute calm. Compared with the distressing existence I had led over those dreadful weeks, I felt as if I had found an oasis of peace and I was so grateful for that. I sat in a soft armchair engulfed in the coloured lights of the tree and my mind suddenly awoke to the fact that I had forgotten it was Christmas!

For the first time I was alone and I didn't cry. I sat and stared into the rainbow of light stretching out from the tree and gathered my thoughts. The house seemed to put its arms around me and enable me to make sense of it all. Indeed Christmas was now only a few days away and I had lost track of that. It felt completely unimportant to me but it meant the world to Jess and somehow, in amongst helping her to face her illness, I would have to try to make Christmas special too. I don't know how long I sat there, but when I decided to move the room was almost completely in darkness apart from the changing lights of the tree. I decided that I would bring Jess to the house the next day, as she would love the peace of that room and the tree, and it would give me the ideal opportunity to talk to her, away from the stress of ward 31.

By the time I had returned to the ward, Jess, along with the other children, had finished tea and she had begun to look for me. She was much brighter in herself now and the soreness caused by her biopsy had eased tremendously, so she was more mobile although still very weak. We chatted for a while about life on the ward and she was obviously taking more notice of the children around her. She began to ask questions about chemotherapy and I explained that this was the treatment for cancer and leukaemia. She could see many children receiving treatment with medicines of all colours and she knew the treatment meant that the children lost their hair. It was evident to me from this conversation that Jess had learned a lot over the previous few days. I had wondered if she just accepted the sad sights of this oncology ward but, on the contrary, I felt she was a stone's throw from asking me what was wrong with her. I knew that once Jess's questions were answered she might begin to make further frightening comparisons with those around her. I was scared for her and wanted to protect her.

Time went by and I helped Jess get ready for bed, drawing the curtain around her for a little privacy in the same way that I had done every night since we had been in Bristol. I pulled up my chair and leant over the side of the bed to cuddle her, and it was then that the inevitable came: "Mummy, what's wrong with me? Why can't we just go home?" My world suddenly stood still; for all of my forward planning, Jess was one step ahead. Slightly shocked, I took a moment to think. My response was always going to be hard no matter when I decided to tell her, but 9.30 p.m. would not be the best time by choice. I thought about all the advice I had been given about being honest with her, and that she was old enough and intelligent enough to be able to deal with the truth.

I took a deep breath and said, "Jess, you know that they were doing some tests following your biopsy last week and it was

37

taking a while for the results to come through. I have known the answer for a while but I wanted you to get your strength back before I told you."

She looked at me with her eyes wide open, unsure of what was coming next. "Before you told me what, Mummy?"

"I'm sorry, Jess, but you've got cancer."

She stared at me in disbelief. "No, no," she repeated over and over, shaking her head with a look of total despair.

I'm not sure what her understanding of cancer was at that stage. I'm sure she realised that it was a nasty illness and she definitely knew that people died from cancer. I decided to tell her everything right from her visit to the hospital in Taunton through to the diagnosis on the previous Friday. I apologised several times for not telling her before and that I had wanted her to recover from the surgery. She held me tightly and sobbed into my shoulder, and in comforting her I knew I would never hide anything from her again. The trust between us would be central to her strength to fight this and be well again. I held her and cried with her, but the relief that I had managed finally to tell her everything was enormous.

On hearing the sound of Jess's desperate sobs, one of the nurses decided to come in and ask what was wrong. I was annoyed at her untimely appearance, more because I wanted to be alone with Jess and it was so hard on this ward to find our own space. She had only the best intentions I am sure, but I snapped something back that made her disappear quicker than she had arrived! I should have been cross with myself really, but I did not allow myself to be distracted from the task in hand. I continued to explain to Jess about the treatment that she would require and that the doctors had decided to start her on her first dose of chemotherapy on Thursday. Jess's consultant had wanted me to talk to her about the side effects of the treatment, which I did, and predictably Jess was very saddened at the thought of losing her hair. She was older than her ten years in so many ways: she was conscious of fashion, her appearance mattered and she was always experimenting with her shoulder-length, thick, light brown hair.

Her next question was possibly the hardest of all to answer. "Am I going to die, Mummy?"

I had been told to be as honest as possible and this proved to be the best advice I was ever given, although sometimes the hardest rule to keep. Again I paused to catch my breath, to allow myself time to think.

"I'm so sorry I couldn't talk to you about all of this sooner, but now you know everything we can work through this together. You have a lot of treatment ahead of you and it's not going to be easy, but I promise I will always be by your side. People can die from cancer and I know you know that, but I will never give up hope, Jess, and I don't want you to either. I will do everything in my power to make sure you won't die, but I can't promise any more than to support you as much as I can. We all love you so much and I will always be here for you. I will never give up on you."

As she hugged me she said, "I love you, Mummy. I promise I won't give up either."

It was understandably really hard for Jess to go to sleep that night. I wished we had spoken earlier in the day, but once she started asking the questions I knew I had to be honest. She cuddled me tightly and I tried hard to comfort her. Laid together on her bed in the middle of this uninviting, overcrowded ward, we had begun our journey together. In the closeness between us she eventually slipped off to sleep. I woke suddenly in the early hours of the morning, stiff from remaining in the same position for hours, and carefully moved away from her side in order to make up my bed on the floor.

Sharing everything with Jess gave me such a sense of relief; a huge weight fell from my shoulders. Suddenly Jess began discussing everything and making her own informed decisions. This was where my hope began. I left all thoughts of death behind and we moved through her treatment step by step. My inspiration came from the other families we met during our time in Bristol. These children showed such immense courage, although not all of them were aware of their individual situations.

Just prior to starting the treatment, Jess was well enough to go to CLIC House and enjoy some peace and quiet with me, a time that we both found uplifting. I was able to cook her favourite food and we could cuddle up on the sofa and enjoy some

Christmas television. When we were there during the daytime, the other families were at the hospital and so we had a very peaceful time. Jess enjoyed the decorations and predictably loved the fibre-optic tree, mesmorised by the dancing rainbow of colour which gently soothed her saddened spirit. It was easy to lose our gaze in the colours, which clearly had a therapeutic effect on both of us. There was a taxi service from the house to the hospital for which I was given vouchers and therefore it was easy to make the journey. During the time that Jess received treatment in Bristol she would always look forward to spending time at CLIC House. If things got tough, this peaceful retreat became almost like a reward to her.

Jess needed a short longline inserting in order for the drugs to be administered (a temporary tube going into a large vein in the arm). Because another anaesthetic was not a good idea, this was done in theatre whilst she was awake. She was incredibly brave and did very well until the surgeon tried to put a stitch through a piece of skin that had not first been numbed. Jess nearly shot through the ceiling, although she was easily calmed afterwards and the team praised her for her bravery. The surgeon that carried out this procedure was really quite a comedian and his sense of humour helped to put Jess at ease. Jess often reminisced about the experience, and although she had many further trips to theatre we sadly never came across him again.

This initial dose of chemotherapy was to last for three days and would be the first of ten. We were informed that these doses would be administered with three-week intervals and that, dependent on blood counts, this regime would continue. It was anticipated that at some stage along the way Jess would travel to Birmingham Children's Hospital to meet Mr de Ville de Goyet for extensive liver surgery, followed by the remaining doses of chemotherapy. This was the great plan that we clung on to through all those weeks of treatment, as having this regime felt safe and gave us confidence about a possible cure. At last, with this first dose, we embarked on a journey feeling as though, after all that Jess had gone through over those previous desperate weeks, we were finally moving towards her ultimate survival.

This first chemotherapy session comprised two drugs, Carboplatin and Cisplatin, which were fed in through her short longline, and at the same time she also received a cocktail of anti-emetic drugs to help her tolerate the treatment and reduce the possible side effect of vomiting. It was a long three days but on the whole she did really well and, although nauseous, she was not actually sick. She slept a great deal and the thought of Christmas kept her going. We were told that once she had finished this chemotherapy session, and as long as she was not being sick, we would be able to go home for Christmas. She was due to finish the treatment on Christmas Eve, so it would be a bit of a rush to get ready but at least we would all be together at home. I must admit the thought of sleeping in a proper bed rather than that filthy floor spurred me on even though I had done precious little throughout the previous weeks to prepare.

Jerzy had been marvellous, working his way through a list of presents for the children and family; he even wrapped everything as well. Jerzy, Gemma and Stewart slept at CLIC House the night before Christmas Eve so that they could be on the ward bright and early for us all to go home together. I think Jess was feeling quite unwell but she would never have admitted that. She was so desperate to go home that she pulled herself together, got dressed and waited patiently in the wheelchair, ready to go the moment her drugs finished. Jess was very strong willed and no doctor was going to stop her going home; she had her heart set on it. We all sat around watching as the last few drops fed through her line, and the relief was so enormous when she was finally allowed to leave. Jess was so happy there were tears of joy in her eyes as we thanked the nurses and pushed her off down the corridor. We were going home for Christmas.

The journey home was uneventful. Jess obviously felt uncomfortable and was glad to lean against me for support. She felt constantly sick and the chemotherapy had made everything taste different. She had been discharged with a huge number of medicines and I would have to get to know what everything was for. All in good time. I felt a bit unsure of how I would cope away from the safety of the hospital. We had not met any of the team in Taunton and with it being Christmas we had been given a telephone number and contact name for the day after Boxing Day. I therefore hoped that all would be okay for the next three days, and I do remember feeling alone with the weight of this new responsibility. Our lives had changed so much in such a short time. I knew I would have to be strong for Jess, but I also had Gemma and Stewart to consider. Jerzy was my tower of strength. I know he felt he had to be strong for me. He said to me later that he felt unable to care for Jess physically, but he could still be there. He said that he loved her dearly but she needed help he could not give and therefore, early on in our journey, he made it his responsibility to look after me so that I could look after Jess. We didn't plan this together, it was just how he saw his role. Jerzy was such a rock to me during that time. Like no other he was able to guide me through and as a result Jess felt secure in the knowledge that we were both pulling together to support her every need.

Finally we arrived home. I remember a feeling of complete relief reaching into my very soul as we rounded the corner and our home came into view. How happy we all were to be back there and together - so simple and perhaps sometimes taken for granted, but now our most significant Christmas wish. Our dog came bounding out to greet us as we helped Jess into the house. She had been weakened by the journey and very soon cuddled up to a pile of cushions on the sofa and drifted off to sleep. She smiled as she slept, and for the first time in weeks I saw her relax into the comfort of familiar surroundings, content that she had made it home for Christmas.

As she slept the rest of us were excitedly rushing around. Gemma and Stewart were beside themselves with the thought of Christmas, running all over the house singing and dancing. I think they had been worried we would not make it home and concerned that Father Christmas might not find us in hospital. They both helped Jerzy put up the decorations and then they all disappeared in search of a Christmas tree and some food for our Christmas dinner. I busied myself clearing up and making ready for Christmas Day. I had done nothing for weeks so there was a lot to do, not to mention washing all the dirty clothes we had bought home.

By the time Jerzy and the children had returned, Jess was still asleep and I had virtually finished the housework. The shelves had been fairly bare in the supermarket but they had managed to find a fair selection of goodies for us and, best of all, Jerzy had bought a fibre-optic tree for Jess. We set about putting it all together and organising the room around this huge tree. We had almost finished when Jess started to stir. As she opened her eyes the room had grown dark and the colours of our new tree reached out to her. She was completely overwhelmed by its beauty and tearfully speechless. The look on her face was thanks enough, but she gave Jerzy an enormous hug. The house now looked entirely different from when we had arrived home. We were all exhausted from the rush but it was definitely worth it. Dinner was organised, the remaining presents were wrapped and we were all finally able to relax and make the best of Christmas together. Jess was so pleased to be home and she loved her tree, the kaleidoscope of colours completing this cosy Christmas scene. We all relaxed in front of the television, and I think I fell asleep for a while, comforted by Jerzy's closeness. I had felt alone in Bristol and now we were all together again.

In our traditional way the children stayed up and enjoyed the anticipation of Christmas Eve. They all eventually went off to bed after putting out a glass of wine and some goodies for Father Christmas and the reindeer. They laid their empty pillowcases at the ends of their beds and settled down to sleep fairly quickly. Jess needed extra cuddles; she wasn't feeling very well following her treatment but clearly she was extremely tired. There was no doubt she needed to sleep, I knew the familiarity and comfort of her own bed would soon overcome her reluctance and do her the world of good. I stayed with her for a while, she whispered her complete joy in being home and her eyes reflected her excitement as she cuddled into me. She was asleep within minutes.

Mum and I went to midnight mass in the same way we had done every year since I was old enough to stay up that late. I felt exhausted and tearful throughout the service and prayed I would be able to carry Jess through all she had to face. I prayed for the bravery I would need to be honest and supportive to her. I remember feeling terrified I would not measure up to all that was required of me. I prayed that God would help, but I never once asked why. Jess's treatment plan was like a journey that was mapped out in front of us. We had to follow this path for her to survive and the regime of treatment in its own way gave us confidence. My dilemma was that Jess depended on me for the strength to continue. I needed to be so much for her and I was scared I would let her down in some way. I sat in that church and prayed for exactly that - the strength to be more than just a mum. I had to carry her gently on her journey, I had promised to be always at her side and I prayed that our closeness would help her find the courage she would need to brave the months of treatment which lay ahead.

Chapter 5

It was gone 8.00 a.m. when Gemma and Stewart woke us. This was late for them, but we had all been so tired the night before and to be quite honest I was glad of the chance to lie in. They excitedly made their way to their presents, delivered by Father Christmas into the conservatory for convenience. Jess had made me promise to wake her so that she could open her presents with Gemma and Stewart. I had not wanted to do this as she looked so peaceful, but I knew how important it was to her so I did as I was told.

She woke up quickly and came downstairs to join the others. It was then that we noticed how the yellowness of her skin had intensified overnight - a worrying development, but we didn't share our concerns. The children worked their way through the gifts, paper flying in all directions, and laughter and excitement taking over for a short while. It was strange for me to watch the presents being opened, as for the first time ever I had not wrapped any of them myself! It was quite exciting to see what they had received. Although I knew what Jerzy and I had decided to get, there were one or two surprises I had not expected. However, the main presents were as we had agreed: Jess had a selection of the latest CDs and a CD player for her bedroom; Gemma had some gymnastic equipment and leotards; and Stewart had a K'nex set. All in all they seemed pleased. I remember thanking Jerzy - if it hadn't been for him they would not have had any presents this year and the disappointment would have been unbearable. I was so grateful he had been able to take care of it all.

Dinner was easily managed. Jerzy had only been able to get hold of a good joint of beef, so there was no stuffing and preparation of that nature to do. Mum had taken care of the vegetables, and as my parents were coming to lunch I knew that Mum would help me serve up. It was only about 10.30 a.m. when Jess went back to bed as she was feeling so tired, and she slept until lunch was ready. She got up and joined in the festivities over our Christmas meal, but was soon asleep again. As distressing as this seemed, she also appeared to be relieved to be at home and so I decided just to continue watching her closely. I knew if we went to the hospital she would be upset. It was a difficult balance between worrying and letting her be. I chose to let her be. She was glad to be at home and I could not find it in my heart to spoil that for her, although we were both desperately worried about her appearance. Apart from Jess sleeping a lot, Christmas Day was a welcome break from the events of the previous week. I remember enjoying a fair amount of alcohol that day - I certainly had a 'floaty' and very relaxed feeling by the end of it!

Boxing Day was relatively the same as Christmas Day, although Jess was becoming progressively more yellow. She slept most of the day away again, but enjoyed a few visitors in between her naps, including Grammy, Grampy (Andrew's mum and dad) and Andrew. It was usual for the children to spend Boxing Day with their dad, but I wanted us to be quiet at home. Jess would not have been well enough to go out anyway. They brought loads of presents from other family members, and Jess was really pleased to see them and enjoyed their visit immensely. They thoughtfully stayed only a short time as Jess was not well, and as they drove off down the road Jess drifted off to sleep again on the sofa. I knew by this point that I would have to contact the hospital first thing in the morning.

Morning came only too quickly and I was relieved finally to make contact with the Children's Unit at Musgrove Park Hospital again. We had been told to contact a Dr Nicky Harris, who would be implementing Jess's treatment in Taunton. Nicky became a very important part of Jessica's story and this was the day we first met. Jess, being tall for her age, was about the same height as Nicky, who struck me as a very professional lady that had a special way with children. Jess immediately took to her. She was kind and gentle when she examined Jess and spent time listening to all Jess had to say. Nicky would discuss things directly with her and avoided talking around her as others had done. Jess enjoyed feeling in control of her treatment and Nicky soon realised this and would talk to us both accordingly.

Jess's bilirubin levels (indicating the severity of her jaundice) had almost doubled, showing that her liver was finding it hard to cope. A CT scan was therefore carried out, which revealed that the tumour had not changed in size. Her liver was noted to be very large and tender. The decreased liver function was thought to be a result of the chemotherapy, which would cause the malignant cells to swell before dying back. It was clear that the treatment had worsened her condition and all we could do was wait and see if things would start to move in a positive direction. She needed medication for the pain and the itching. Sleeping at night for long periods of time was difficult and this was why she seemed happier to sleep intermittently through the day. It was around this time that we got into the habit of allowing Jess to stay up late with Jerzy and I, thus shortening the length of time she had to be alone at night. She felt confident sleeping in the daytime when she had people around her. Jess also enjoyed the chance to spend long periods of uninterrupted time with us whilst Gemma and Stewart were in bed. We enjoyed playing board games together. She loved Cluedo and a horse-racing game that involved basic principles of betting. Battleships was another favourite - blowing up boats seemed to relieve some anger and frustration for her! Looking back on these few weeks, I know now how close Jess was to not making it through. Her liver was effectively failing, but I only learned this much later in her journey.

After a couple of weeks Jess's hair started to fall out, as predicted. It did so gradually and was almost unnoticeable at first. This was the most distressing symptom for Jess, she was at an age where her developing image was crucial to her self esteem and she hated the thought of not having any hair. She was worried her friends would make fun of her and she was scared of rejection. I took her out in her wheelchair to have a look round the sales and we were able to buy a wide array of hats in all colours and designs. She had a fun time trying them on and Gemma and Stewart joined in, and we laughed at some of the truly awful ones they managed to find. Jess's brother and sister were somehow able to help make light of the situation and help Jess to break free from her more serious inhibitions. They obviously had no idea that their fun-filled attitudes were helping me so much, but the truth was that in these early days they were vital in helping Jess to want to live on. Without their spurring her on in their humorous way, she would have found each hurdle far more difficult.

On most days we were visited by someone from the hospital. Often either Nicky or one of the community oncology nurses (known as CLIC nurses) would come to the house to keep a close eye on how Jess was doing. On the whole I felt there were improvements and a blood test on 2 January 2001 proved me right. She was still jaundiced but her bilirubin levels had definitely improved. We still had a long way to go, but this meant she would be fit enough to return to Bristol Children's Hospital the following day for further chemotherapy. Because Jess's first dose of treatment had caused her liver huge problems, we would have to stay at the hospital for longer this time in case her situation became worse again. They had decided to use a different drug this time, Doxorubicin, and there was concern as to how her body would react to it. The plan was to alternate this drug with the first regime throughout her ten treatments. The intention would be to discharge her to CLIC House rather than back home so that we would be close to the ward if further problems occurred.

So Jess and I packed to leave home again. We were more organised this time and committed to our journey together. Stewart and Gemma were returning to school and I had confidence in Jerzy and my mum to take care of them. However, I felt as though we had all just managed to settle back into home life again. We had achieved a level of happiness over the Christmas holiday and now it was all changing. I hated leaving but we had no choice, we had to travel this road together no matter how hard it was. Jess was sad not to be returning to school and she worried continuously about her SATs and falling behind.

When we arrived back on the ward at Bristol we found many of the same families there, so it didn't feel as daunting as our first visit and it was great to be able to continue the friendships we had made. Jess was scheduled for surgery the next day to insert a Hickman line (a more permanent flexible tube passing through the side of her chest directly into the large veins near her heart), through which her chemotherapy could be administered more easily. Her short longline had become very uncomfortable and had a tendency to catch on everything, so she was glad to be having it removed. The Hickman line would make life easier for her and would hopefully prove to be less of an irritation. Once inserted, the nursing staff would immediately set about administering her next dose of chemotherapy.

The operation went well and she recovered quickly from the anaesthetic. It was not such a complex operation as her biopsy, and although she was a little sore this soon passed. She was able to enjoy the company of her new-found friends more fully than before. As school had started again, the teachers had returned to the ward, which Jess found delightful. She enjoyed the tasks that were set for her and some of the displays, such as a fishy collage for the wall, and I enjoyed joining in as well. I would read to her when she was tired and she had brought a selection of videos, knowing she would have her own TV to watch. The chemotherapy went well and she seemed to sleep more comfortably than before. Again she was put on strong drugs to limit her sickness, which seemed to do the trick. After three days we were discharged, as promised, to CLIC House where we were able to enjoy some home cooking again and a special kind of peace away from the ward. Following her discharge, however, Jess suddenly became tired, she had a horrible taste in her mouth making it hard for her to eat and she became quite unwell.

Sarah and Steve drove up to see us with the children, which provided welcome light relief and Jess was thrilled to see her friends. They played happily together, although I could see that Jess was struggling. Katie had been given a cuddly toy that gave birth to babies if you made a big fuss of it! This kept the children amused for ages and I welcomed the opportunity to speak to Sarah and Steve. Later, after our friends had left, Jess was not well at all. She was in severe pain and asked to go back to the hospital. As her distress grew the taxi seemed to take ages, when finally we arrived on the ward she was in agony and was re-admitted for pain control and a scan was booked to see what was going on. She looked awful and said very little. She was disappointed by her physical decline after having such a wonderful time with her friends. We were both tearful, although I did my best to comfort her with the thought of her feeling slightly better tomorrow. Her blood results had again worsened and I was told it might be necessary to insert some kind of stent to relieve the pressure on her bile duct.

The MRI scan revealed the tumour was not shrinking, although on a positive note it had not progressed either. Despite this mixed news it was not possible to insert a stent. Mr Spicer came to see me and whilst Jess slept he explained why the operation would not be appropriate in Jess's case. The tumour remained inoperable and therefore there was little more that could be done. If the chemotherapy did not start to reduce the tumour, Jess would become progressively weaker. She slept for what seemed like days, whilst I stayed by her side and watched over her, willing her to start showing some kind of improvement.

At last her blood results started to improve and she gradually became more wakeful. What a relief, and what a roller-coaster this journey seemed to be. Just as things started to look better, they would become worse; and just when you thought it was all nearly over, she would improve again. I was exhausted but relieved that for the moment we were on the up. At last we were able to return home, much to the delight of Jess and her brother and sister. Again we rejoiced that we were once more reunited.

Our joy, however, only lasted a couple of days, as suddenly Jess became neutropenic. I had been warned about this, but we were about to experience the effects of it first hand. It meant, in very basic terms, that Jess's immune system had been suppressed and she was now susceptible to infections of all kinds. Even the simplest of bugs that live on our skin on a day-to-day basis can become a source of infection for children who are neutropenic. We had been told that the first signs of trouble would be a dramatic increase in temperature. This came over Jess all of a sudden and she needed to be admitted to hospital straight away for investigation of the bug and intravenous antibiotics to control the problem. The investigations into her infection revealed that she needed to be given a specific antibiotic called Teicoplanin. Jess had been busily taking part in some papier mâché that day - we were making an elephant by covering a balloon with sticky paper and Jess had planned to decorate it during a later visit. Creating this elephant had become an immensely enjoyable project for her.

We broke off from this activity for a moment whilst the new antibiotic was given to Jess, as it was administered through her hickman line she developed a sudden and severe reaction to it. She gasped for air and cried out through her shortened breath, "Mummy, I'm dying, Mummy, Mummy!" Her lips turned blue and she became very nauseous. Someone ran to get Nicky, who immediately gave Jess a hydrocortisone injection along with some piriton for good measure. Over the course of the afternoon Jess's symptoms settled down, but the experience had frightened her and she understandably became very wary of what medicine was being given to her after that. 'Teicoplanin' was then written on all of Jess's notes in big red letters to alert all medical staff of her severe allergy to it. The experience had been a bit of a scare for everyone.

This stay in hospital turned out to be a long one. Jess had her antibiotics, then she had a blood transfusion and a platelet infusion and finally it was full steam ahead for the third dose of chemotherapy. As this dose was due to be Cisplatin again, Jess's oncologist in Bristol was happy to allow her to have the treatment at Taunton rather than going to Bristol again. This was marvellous news. It meant that the children could visit and I would be able to nip home from time to time. She was able to take more things with her, including her own music, duvet and pillows, and was allocated her own isolated cubicle, a more personal space than available on the ward in Bristol. And, instead of sleeping on the floor, I now had a sofa bed in the same cubicle, which made life more comfortable for me.

However, despite our improved hospital experience, by the time we reached the third day of chemotherapy Jess had become very depressed and anxious that she was going to die. This was apparently one of the side effects of a drug she had to take during chemotherapy to keep her from being ill. I always knew, however, that once we were home it would not be long before her spirits would inflate again. It was during these low ebbs that Jess's fears would come to the surface and I had to work hard to reassure and comfort her. She would sleep a lot and not want to see anyone, her patience with Gemma and Stewart would become shortened and her abruptness would lead to arguments. During these times it became easier to keep them all apart, although this was harder on me because I then found myself torn in two. By the time this third session of treatment was over I felt incredibly relieved to be going home, as Jess's physical and emotional needs were taking their toll on me and I needed to recharge my batteries.

It was encouraging, though, that Jess's blood results had shown a great improvement and her large, tender liver seemed to be diminishing in size. Despite the ups and downs of the journey, we were making definite progress. I was able to talk to Jess about this and remind her of how far she had come when she got down. The treatment seemed relentless to her and, despite her answers to the doctors, she would talk quite openly to me about dying. She definitely saw her future as being short-lived. She found it hard to tolerate visitors, as she worried about her appearance and being rejected. She was unsure about ever going to school again and dreaded the reaction of her friends to her physical changes. She had gained weight quickly, due in part to the steroids she was on. Almost all her hair had fallen away apart from a wispy fringe. Although she visibly looked more well than she had in ages, she did look different and she was very conscious of this.

It was around this time that Jess met her home tutor for the first time. It was a scary experience for Jess as, although she enjoyed learning, she had missed so much school by this time. As we eagerly awaited the tutor's arrival Jess was clearly nervous. I had helped her with her reading and we had done various artistic projects at home, but it had been months since she had had any formal education. Finally her tutor breezed in. She possessed a bright and bubbly disposition, was confident in her manner and, importantly for Jessica, she did not react to her appearance. They quickly became friends and we arranged for her to visit for about an hour a day. They worked on French, English and Maths and discussed the books that Jess had read. Throughout Jess's treatment, when she was too ill to do anything, I would read to her. She liked to hear the sound of my voice, and focusing on a story helped her to feel less alone and allowed her mind to travel to a different place. Her tutor helped to fuel Jess's need for artistic stimulation and would come up with all sorts of different things for her to do. She was a lovely person to have around and she really helped Jess to develop her potential. She quickly realised how clever Jess was and worked very much to her ability. Some days following treatment Jess could do little more than lie on the sofa, but her tutor understood this and would bring a game to play rather than formal work of any kind. She learned to get the most from Jess on the occasions when she was up to applying herself.

Gradually, as her condition improved, Jess would try to get to school for the odd afternoon. She was initially most conscious of her hair, the last of which was still falling out. She wore a hat to try to contain it but got very upset if any fell on the desk in front of her. When this happened she felt as if everyone had seen it and became incredibly embarrassed, even though in truth I doubt anyone had noticed. She had also required the wheelchair at times, as initially the treatment had weakened her and she sometimes needed the additional support. I went to the school and spoke to the head, who was always very keen to help wherever he could. I explained how upset Jess was over her hair and how she felt about her appearance. The next day a whole host of letters and cards arrived from school. Everyone had written to Jess to tell her how much they missed her and that they were not worried about how she appeared. The older year-six students, Jess's closer friends, had made a tape recording of her favourite music. They talked to her about how brilliant she was, a good friend whom they missed very much. I sat and listened to the tape with her, and she was quite touched by it. Then she said, "That's it, Mummy, I am definitely going to school tomorrow!"

This was a big turning point for Jess, as now she was able to go to school and enjoy her friends' company again. The small family environment of the school meant she held the friendship of children of all ages and their good wishes helped to carry her through.

And so we went through this cycle of treatment every three weeks, followed by initial illness and then gradual improvement, at which point she would be having home tuition as well as attending school for the afternoon. However, just as things started to feel much improved, we would be back at the hospital for more chemotherapy. It was a seemingly endless cycle, but we took each step one at a time. We were spurred on by the good times and found the strength between us to navigate the sad times. The highs came with good blood or scan results; the lows with neutropenia, blood transfusions and chemotherapy. Overall, by the end of February 2001, it was very clear that Jess was doing really well. Her jaundice had subsided, the tumour had shrunk to half its original size and she was gradually regaining her strength.

Sarah and all four of her children were performing in *Babes in the Wood*, a pantomime that Jess had long looked forward to. The hospital managed to finish her chemo just in time and she was able to enjoy the performance. After everything that had happened, Jess was thrilled to be able to enjoy this show. She had set her heart on being there and it gave her the inspiration to push on and be well enough. I remember being slightly ill at ease during that performance, as Gemma's seat was right next to the Mayor and Mayoress. However, she behaved wonderfully and I was very proud of her, although a little anxious at times! This was an evening of total enjoyment and I felt as though we were back to being an ordinary family again just having fun. We were all in the front row and I enjoyed heckling Sarah who played the wicked queen. I think she has forgiven me now!

Anyone who has experienced a chemotherapy regime for themselves or alongside a child will know just how exhausting a treatment it is. By March we were ready for a break and a holiday flat was offered to us at Sidmouth. The flat belonged to CLIC and was provided for families such as ours to enjoy a break away from home. The accommodation was completely free and we were allocated a five-day break. I remember the weather was dreadful - unfortunately very cold and wet. The flat was right on the seafront and the children enjoyed watching the thunderous waves beating against the sea wall. The accommodation, however, was cosy and warm, there were freshly baked cakes waiting for us when we arrived and the peace of being away from the telephone for a few days was bliss. This was a very special few days for us all as a family. Gemma and Stewart had some wonderful toys to play with and there were family games of all kinds, so when the weather was really bad we played games and enjoyed our own company. When the rain eased we went for short walks on the beach or took Jess around the shops in a wheelchair. She found the pebbled beach hard to walk on but the fresh air was invigorating.

Sidmouth has some lovely individual gift shops and Jess spent ages planning what she was going to buy. She spent much of her money on presents for people, mainly her school friends, and very little on herself. Gemma and Stewart, however, were intent on spending their money on whatever they could. This was a sign to me that Jess had grown up very much over those last few months, as there was a time when money would have burnt a hole in her pocket but not anymore. She demonstrated to me how sensible she had become. I even remember her beginning to protect me from her brother and sister when they constantly asked for further money to spend.

Jess had become such a companion to me, and the amount of time we had spent in each other's company had led our relationship to another level. We would talk as good friends and laugh together, and she shared how she felt in a way that she was never able to do with anyone else. She trusted in my strength and yet she had grown stronger emotionally than she realised. She had found her own inner confidence being totally commited to this journey and ultimately the hope of survival. This trip was a remarkable few days, a chance to take stock of just how far Jess had come and return a little revived, ready to take on the next phase of her treatment. Jess had shown immense courage and gradually she had matured beyond her years. Perhaps it was the honesty we shared that informed her awareness of self, but she had changed immeasurably, especially over those first few months of treatment. It wasn't just a physical change; an internal shift took place as well. She grew in determination whilst keeping a sense of grace and dignity. It was easy to see how many of her school friends came to look up to her and so many, touched by her story, admired her for her strength.

Chapter 6

We had already sat for almost three hours, alone in a parents' lounge, staring at the cracks in the wall or the well-used furniture. We had run out of conversation and every ounce of my body was shaking with fear. Surely someone should know something by now?

Jerzy and I had accompanied Jess to theatre at just gone 8.30 a.m. and she had been anaesthetised at 8.50 a.m. We had said our goodbyes as the team of theatre staff at Birmingham Children's Hospital waited to take charge of her. I cuddled her, held her hand and then kissed her gently as she closed her eyes and sank into enforced sleep. "Take care of her for me," I had said simply, the tears running down my face as Jerzy and I were led out into the corridor. We stood, holding each other and crying together, for some while before we were escorted back to ward 10. We were both so scared. We had tried to be positive for Jess's sake, but we knew that Mr de Ville de Goyet and his team had a long day ahead of them and we would have very little idea of what was happening.

The ward staff gave us a bleeper so that we could wander off and take in some fresh air. However, this did not give me any sense of security and I could not bear to be far from her, so we chose to sit in the nearest seating area to the theatre and I would not leave. I was constantly hoping that we would be told what was happening. The day before, we had met Mr de Ville de Goyet for only the second time. His tall, commanding presence and wonderful French accent had made an instant impression on me. All his team seemed to hold him in reverence and he was clearly very well respected in his field. Jess liked him too. He explained in detail what he intended to do and drew some pictures so that she was fully aware of her situation. He explained how the tumour was sitting very close to the portal vein and that he was unsure whether he would be able to remove it or not. He wanted Jess to understand it might not be possible and he may only be able to stitch her back up again without attempting to remove the tumour. Although there had initially been significant shrinkage, thereafter the tumour had remained a constant size despite large amounts of chemotherapy. Nobody knew whether the tumour was now simply dead tissue and had been suppressed successfully by the chemotherapy or whether the treatment had just held the cancer at bay for the duration and it was waiting to spring into action once her treatment had finished. A lot of the questions we all had would be answered today, although it was clear that Jess was going to have a tough time. Mr de Ville de Goyet had told us that it would be a difficult operation to perform, even if it were a technical success there was a strong chance Jess could go into liver failure in the few days following the procedure. If the latter, we would then be reliant on an emergency liver transplant.

Jess had sat bravely and listened to all he had to say and she was fully aware of all that rested on the outcome of that day. She knew that she could not survive unless the tumour were removed, but she also knew the risks of the surgery and the possibility that she might bleed extensively. This amazing man had explained how difficult it was to dissect the liver because it was so full of blood vessels. We were putting so much faith in him; we had to believe he could do it.

After a lengthy conversation with Mr de Ville de Goyet and his team I was handed the consent form to complete and sign. I turned to Jess and said, "Have you understood everything, Jess? Is this what you want to do?" She replied confidently, "I know I won't get better unless we try this. I want to do it, Mummy." I knew I would have to be the one to sign the form, but I had worried about how I would feel if she didn't make it. I had signed a few forms for the other small procedures, but this was major. We knew the odds were that she could die in surgery or soon afterwards and I worried that I would feel as though I had signed her life away. She convinced me that this was what she wanted and for her sake we had to follow this path. I took a deep breath and then signed the form. I didn't know how I would survive while she was in theatre, I was so afraid for her, but she was so together and strong. Her courage was incomparable, her bravery unsurpassed. That evening she had said she just wanted to get on with it now; the waiting had been

57

hard for her to bear.

We had been told that the decision would be made once they had opened her up. Three hours had comfortably gone by and there was still no word, so I felt confident that the surgery must have continued. We decided to go back to the ward and ask one of the nurses if they could find out anything, Five hours had been mentioned as a maximum for the procedure, so I concluded that he must have found he could continue.

We waited patiently for the call to be made and then the news came that Mr de Ville de Goyet had still not decided if he could do it. Three hours and no decision. It must have been a tough one to make, and he had said that once he had made the decision to go for it there would be no going back. We were reassured that Jess was fine and that she was having no problems coping with the anaesthetic. Still unable to leave, we returned to the parents' lounge and cuddled up on the sofa, completely bewildered that she had been in theatre for so long and yet they had not reached a decision.

I lost myself in memories, wonderful memories of my beautiful child. I remembered her birth, the first time I held her. She was a perfect baby: 9lb 3½ oz of pure joy. As she was my first child I had a lot to learn, but she was so much fun. Dimples used to appear on her cheeks when she smiled and from a very early age she had such a hearty laugh. I remembered her taking her first steps and how when she fell over she could not get herself up again! Her first pair of shoes had been made of pink canvas and she was so proud of them. She had a radiant complexion and a perfect face with sparkling blue eyes. She had always been taller than her peers and I imagined that she would be very tall when she grew up. I now prayed that she would have the chance to grow up.

I remembered when she started playschool and how I collected all her pictures and pinned them to the back of the kitchen door. I had painted a picture of Postman Pat on one wall of her bedroom and Mickey Mouse, Minnie Mouse and Pluto on the other. We lived in a lovely cottage in Wiveliscombe then. It was small and cosy and we had a log burner for heating during the winter months. We had been happy there and Jess always remembered that house fondly. It was here that she made a snowman one winter; the snow never seemed to fall as it did when I was a child. It was as tall as her shoulders when we had finished and wore an old hat and scarf. We used a carrot for its nose and some glass pebbles for its eyes, mouth and the buttons down the front. She had loved this snowman and often mentioned it. By this time Gemma had been born and Jess loved having a baby sister. Stewart arrived 14 months later and we moved house, and things were never quite the same again. Jess often talked about our first home; we had many happy memories in that house. I smiled to myself as I thought of those days again.

Jess had enjoyed helping to care for Stewart. She was four years old when he was born and loved to help bath and look after him. Stewart grew up especially close to Jess; she did everything for him and they had a very special affinity. Gemma was always mischievous. She had a lively spirit about her, always up to something and never standing still for a minute. Her behaviour would agitate Jess and it was sometimes hard to keep the peace. It was normal sisterly behaviour no doubt, and they loved each other really, but it was so refreshing when there was peace between them.

Jess started attending Milverton Primary School. I remembered having a broken ankle at the time. Jess enjoyed the excitement of her new school; she was confident and made many friends. She loved a challenge and developed some wonderful personal qualities that would set her up well for the future. As for me, I found life difficult at our new house. We were struggling financially and I took a job working for a local supermarket, stacking shelves and monitoring the stock on the computer system. I would go to work at about 7.30 p.m. and come home sometimes as late as 2.00 a.m. or 3.00 a.m. the following morning. I remembered how tired I had been driving in every night and the drive home would be awful as well. I found it hard to keep my eyes open, my eyelids would be heavy with sleep and there would be moments of lost consciousness and panic to keep the car on the road. Consequently, I was always tired, and taking care of three young children on top of very little sleep was hard work. Later on I started my own face-painting business, which took me all over the place. Sometimes

I travelled many miles to attend shows and I worked for large shops for promotional purposes. We desperately needed extra money at this time and through my little business I had hoped to help bring in enough to make the difference. Perhaps it was naive to think I could make that much of a difference, but it is always so easy in hindsight to realise your own mistakes. The truth was that it took me away from my children on days when I would rather have been at home. The business cost me more than I had anticipated and it caused a huge amount of stress, adding to our financial worries at the time. My marriage to Andrew fell irreparably apart and I decided not to continue with the face painting. I wanted to be with the children, to be the best mum I could, and I faced up to my own mistakes. I took a job with a local newspaper and by working full-time my wage was just enough to purchase a 50 per cent share in a housing association house. Inwardly I felt lost and alone with my three children; few friends had stuck by me and my self-esteem was at an almighty low. My little business had failed alongside my marriage and I wondered how I would ever survive this time. It was hard but we were happy together and the children were amazing. Gradually they had each helped me unknowingly to repair my soul.

Our new house was lovely, and as it was situated opposite my mum and dad the children enjoyed being close to their grandma and grandad. I enjoyed the emotional support they were able to offer at the time and my mum helped me endlessly to care for the children. She would take the children to school and collect them at the end of the day for me, tirelessly helping with anything she could. This constant support was priceless, providing much-needed continuity for the children whilst I worked as hard as I could to keep us all. The move had brought a change of school for Jessica and Gemma, and Stewart was just starting school so I was able to introduce him to Nynehead from the beginning. Nynehead was my childhood home and fond memories surrounded this unspoilt village, so introducing the children to the primary school was like returning home for me. Including my three children, the numbers attending the school only reached about 21, so I think the school was glad at the time to boost the numbers! The children settled into their new environment immediately, never asking questions but just accepting life as it was. They all grew in confidence and I was so proud of them all, but Jess in particular, being the eldest, had been an amazing strength to me. She was wonderful company and so mature and responsible for her age. We all pulled together and very soon started to enjoy life together again. We enjoyed simple pastimes that didn't cost money, such as cycling or walking, flying kites, picnics and the seaside.

"Would you like me to try to find a sandwich and a drink?" Jerzy woke me from my daydream. It was 1.30 p.m. and there was still no further news. "I think we should have something to eat. You had no breakfast so you should have something. I'll find some food and then we'll see if there is any more news."

I nodded. I was unable to have sensible conversation; every time we spoke tears would trickle down my face. This day was dreadful and every minute felt like an eternity. I couldn't do anything. I was unable to read, watch television or even go for a walk. All I could do was lose myself in my thoughts. It wasn't long before Jerzy returned with some food from the shop at the entrance, I felt sick but he was right, as always - I needed to keep my strength up to care for Jess.

By 2.00 p.m. she had been under anaesthetic for five hours, so we decided to go back to the ward to see if there was any news. We waited and waited for the nurse to return from her call to theatre. Again she told us that Jess was fine and there was no need to worry but Mr de Ville de Goyet had started to remove the tumour and the message was that they were expecting to be in theatre for a long time. That was it; he was doing it and there would be no going back now. I started to shake again. I was glad he was having a go but at what cost? There were so many risks involved. As I walked away from ward 10 the fear returned and my tears flowed uncontrollably.

I headed for the chapel, which was just across the corridor from where Jess lay in theatre. I needed to be close to her but I wanted to pray. The knowledge that there was no going back echoed around in my mind. I prayed that God would guide the surgeon's hand and bring my beautiful child through. I was so scared, I didn't know what to do with myself, and I felt so helpless. Jerzy went to telephone the family and left me alone in the chapel. I needed to be quiet and I was happy to be left alone. It was a very peaceful place, completely lined with marble and with the most wonderful stained-glass windows. There was such a complete contrast when you walked into the chapel from the busy corridor outside and met with the silence of that place. The heavy stone walls kept back the noise of the hospital and allowed the atmosphere to be filled with peace and serenity. I sat numbed by the news. My head was hurting from crying and my face felt sore from constantly being wet with tears. I looked around me and stared at everything and yet at nothing at all. My gaze eventually fixed on one of the splendid windows and I drifted into my memories again.

Nynehead village church had beautiful windows and was full of character and charm. I remembered the services that had been held there by the school. Jess had enjoyed playing the recorder and singing as required, always prepared to be involved where necessary. The Christmas before she became ill Jess had played the angel Gabriel in church and had looked very ethereal in her lacy costume and wings. She had presented herself with such pride in front of her audience. Gemma was one of her many angels and Stewart, who was very young and whose acting skills had not fully developed, was a shepherd. Jess had laughed so much watching Stewart walking off round the church pointing at an imaginary star in the sky with a teacloth on his head! Jess had the commanding role and as always she pulled it off to perfection.

Christmas was my favourite time - the children so loved Christmas and their excitement was infectious. Every year on Christmas Eve I would put straw around the house, little bits here and there, as though Father Christmas had trodden all over the house. I would put reindeer food down as well and make believe that this was what made the reindeer fly. Jess used to call the reindeer food 'magic oats'. The glass of brandy along with the sweets and mince pies would be gone, and only a little evidence of the carrots for the reindeer would remain for the children to find in the morning. It worked every year: the children were always totally convinced that Father Christmas had really been in the house. It was then customary to make a fuss when clearing up the mess. I had to be cross that he had trodden all over the house with dirty boots. Jess would stand up for him, saying, "He's really busy, Mummy, he doesn't have time to wipe his feet!" I smiled to myself as I remembered how she carried on the story for Gemma and Stewart even when she had realised the truth herself. Christmas was always a magic time for them. To believe in something so magical is lovely, and this simplicity is so often lost in today's commercial world.

Jerzy returned with good wishes sent from friends and family. It felt as though everyone was holding their breath, waiting on each phone call, afraid to move away from the phone just as we were afraid to go far from Jess. Andrew was sitting outside. I felt sorry for him, but my own fears did not leave room for comforting him as well. He had arrived at the hospital after Jess had gone into theatre and therefore had not been able to wish her well. His girlfriend was with him, so he did have someone he could lean on. I had asked not to meet her that day. I was in such a state and we had not met before, so this did not seem the right time, although I always wished them well. Therefore he sat outside where they could be alone together and every so often we would arrange to meet back at the ward for an update. The next update came at 4.00 p.m.. Jess was all right but they felt the procedure would take another hour or so. Every minute was painful to me; she had now been gone for seven hours. Although Mr de Ville de Goyet had explained that it could be a difficult operation, I had not realised just how complex this surgery must be for it to take so long.

We remained in the chapel together for a while. Jerzy was as glad to drink in the peace that this special place offered as I was. He was so supportive and his love for Jess was obvious. He cared for her as a daughter and she had come to love him as another father. All the children accepted Jerzy for the different qualities he brought to their lives. He was a computer programmer from London who after being made redundant had become a driving instructor. Jerzy was a mine of information and knew so much across a wide variety of subjects. He had enjoyed maths at school and was able to work through the most complex of problems. His computer knowledge was invaluable and he was always ready to help the children with projects and topics of all kinds. His thirst for knowledge was infectious, providing a wonderful example for the children. He encouraged them to quest for information and he would help them to answer their own questions, and above all he loved music. The first time he met Jess she had asked him to help her load a French programme onto my computer, and he sat and patiently helped her to achieve her aim, instantly winning her over. It wasn't hard to love him, and the children had found it easy. He was big, tall and cuddly, but most of all he always wore a smile. He was laid back and never seemed to get flustered; he had a strong and stable disposition, always kind, gentle and caring. He stood by me, holding me up when I felt weak and encouraging me when I was unsure. He taught me to believe in myself again when I was alone and lost. Jerzy had become my right hand and I could not imagine life without him.

I remembered how Jerzy would take the children to school for me in the mornings and how he had taught them to sing "We don't need no education" as they went off in the car! They found this very amusing; I just hoped they didn't continue to sing it at school. I also remembered our bicycle rides before Jess had become ill. We would pack up a picnic and ride the bikes down to this spot we knew on the river. Jerzy had bought a bike with too many gears and he would lose his balance and cycle into the hedge every time he tried to change a gear. Jess found this a hilarious quality; although she often tried to help him it never seemed to make a difference. Our dog, Jet, would run alongside, although she soon learned to stay close to me, knowing that the space around Jerzy's bike was not a safe place to be. The children would play in the river and we would tuck into our picnic - a simple family pleasure and one that we all enjoyed tremendously.

As we sat together quietly in the chapel I cuddled up to Jerzy for comfort. I was so grateful that he was there to lean on. How would I have managed to cope with all this alone? We made our way back to the parents' lounge again, with another hour still to go until our next update was due at 6.00 p.m. Judging from our last message, hopefully Jess would be emerging from theatre by then. We would then have reached the nine-hour mark, when they surely must be nearly finished.

I remembered Jess's bravery and her faith in God; she trusted in his strength to help her through. She had found the months of chemotherapy hard, and her troubled life had suddenly brought her closer to her faith. She had asked to be confirmed and along with her friend Kylie she had taken her first communion. This had not been something she was pushed into as with so many children whose parents' expectations lead them along this path. The magical thing was that her life suddenly filled with the love of Christ and she chose to acknowledge her belief by asking to be confirmed. The ceremony took place during the week prior to her eleventh birthday. Bishop Andrew struck me as one of the most amazing men I have ever met. He was hilariously full of fun and the service was made an absolute joy by his ability to capture the attention of his congregation. He often talked about Jess after the event; he was touched by her courage and her genuine love of Christ. She had asked if it was all right to wear a hat as she had very little hair at the time, and he had explained that a hat would not stop the Holy Spirit, but when the time came she removed it anyway! Now that she was able to take communion she would comment regularly on the wine. If it had been snatched away a bit too quickly she would complain that she had not managed to take a large enough sip! She was so pleased to show her faith in God and her trust in the Lord was a strong guiding force in helping her to face life through the difficult times ahead. I prayed that our Lord would hear our prayer, then surely she would survive.

Following her confirmation at the weekend we celebrated her eleventh birthday by throwing a huge party for her. We invited the whole school, teachers as well as pupils, plus friends and family. We had organised a disco and there was enough food to feed an army. Sarah and her girls had worked tirelessly on a banner that read 'Happy Birthday Jessica', which was hung from the ceiling along with hundreds of balloons and other decorations. The disco man had arrived with a karaoke machine. Jess was initially unsure about this, but once it was set up the children argued continuously over who would be the next to go up and sing. Jess thoroughly enjoyed herself and we found it difficult to pull her away to cut her cake, as she was more worried about losing her place in the queue. We had organised team games, helped along by my cousin Graham who always had an idea up his sleeve. We knew this could possibly be her last birthday and I wanted her to know how much we all loved her - and she did.

The minutes that had seemed like hours had slowed even more, but 6.00 p.m. eventually came. Jerzy and I were completely drained by the emotional turmoil of the day. Surely there would be news? They couldn't possibly tell us to go away for another two hours. This time Andrew did not turn up, as he had gone to find something to eat. We were told that she was still in theatre and that they had decided she would not be brought back to ward 10 but would remain in intensive care so that she could be monitored more closely. Mr de Ville de Goyet had sent the message that they would not be much longer and that we should wait in intensive care for her to come out of theatre. We were warned that they had decided to keep Jess on the ventilator and not wake her up for a while as she had had such a long operation. Exhausted, bewildered and scared, we followed the nurse along the corridor towards intensive care. She was going to show us around, to familiarise us as far as possible with what to expect. The truth was I didn't know what to expect; since Jessica had first become ill I had gradually learned not to expect anything but to go with and cope with things as they were. This philosophy had worked well up to now but I was still shaking with fear, as I had done all day. I just wanted my little girl back. I had been on the ward early to help prepare Jess for theatre and those last couple of hours with her had been hard for Jess as well as for me. She was nervous and just wanted to get on with it. I tried hard to get her ready confidently, never letting it show for a minute how I felt inside. Then we had said goodbye and now nine hours later we were on our way to intensive care hoping that at last we would see her again. It had been a long day but it was far from over yet. As I walked briskly up the corridor hand in hand with Jerzy, I just prayed she would be all right.

Chapter 7

Intensive care was huge, reminding me of an airport, although clinically clean as you might expect. This vast expanse of white space was a daunting experience and perhaps this was why they had wanted to show us around now rather than later, as it took some getting used to. Despite the vastness there were very few beds and we were shown to the 'station' that had been allocated to Jess. As there was no bed present at the time we were merely shown yet another space, the only difference being the bridge of monitors and machines that arched over it. I was truly daunted by all the machinery, but the most important part they wanted to impress upon us was that she would still be on a ventilator on arrival from theatre. They were worried how I was going to react. I looked such a state from crying all day that I'm not surprised they were worried. I reassured them that I would just be so pleased to see her again.

We were then shown to another waiting room within the confines of intensive care, which was positioned right beside the lift that would bring Jess down from theatre. Knowing this meant that we were constantly looking every time the lift door opened to see if it was Jess. Andrew caught up with us eventually and waited a while, but there was still no news and he had to catch a train back to his brother's house and could not wait any longer. I know he wanted to stay and he was very sad that he had missed her before and now would not see her until tomorrow. Jerzy and I continued to wait in the hope that soon there would be some indication of how she was getting on. One of the nurses brought me some paracetamol for my headache, which I duly took, and then I tried to rest my head and close my eyes to relieve the pain. Not asleep but consumed in thought I tried to rest, waiting pensively as ever.

We had known for a long time that this operation would be difficult. This was why we had given Jess such a huge party for her eleventh birthday. I wanted her to know how much everyone loved her and that we were all willing her to get through. As a run-up to this trip to Birmingham I had suggested that Jess should make a wish list: a list of things she most wanted to do before she went into hospital. Her first wish was to paddle in the sea. As already mentioned, Jess loved the water, but as there had been a risk of infection due to the chemotherapy regime suppressing her immune system we had stayed away from the seaside. Just before the operation, however, she had not had treatment for a number of weeks and her immunity had picked up considerably. I therefore decided to risk it.

What a memorable day we had. We met up with Sarah and her four girls and we all headed off to Charmouth. I taped a plastic sandwich bag over Jessica's Hickman line to try to protect it from splashes of water and the sand. She played all day in the sea, coming very close to submerging her line under the seawater on occasions, which would not have been a good idea. It must have been hard for her but she clearly enjoyed herself so much. They had water fights, chased around and tried to catch Sarah and I out on occasions with the odd bucket of water. We took a lovely picnic and just enjoyed a thoroughly wonderful day. The sun shone constantly and later, when we had had enough of the beach, we took a kite up on the hill and the children took turns to fly it in the sea breeze. They all worked together to keep it high in the sky until Stewart took charge and lost control - a gust of wind took it from his hands and it flew into the next field. All seven children followed after it in dismay. However, we were unable to reach it as our path was blocked by a hedge thick with stinging nettles. Fortunately, two boys had seen our plight and decided to help, managing to catch the kite and return it to us, much to the relief of Stewart who was beside himself as he had been the one who had let it go.

We continued to walk along the beach looking for fossils in the late afternoon sun. Here they all were, all seven happily enjoying their day, glad to have each other's friendship and to share this special time together. We walked in and out of the waves breaking gently on the shore, searching for anything that looked prehistoric. Sometimes the odd shapes of the stones would lead us to believe we had found an amazing fossil of some kind, although it was more likely just a coloured rock worn down by years of tossing in the sea. They were all happy to believe in what we had found, however, and went home with plenty of relics to remember our day by. They all knew the difficulties that Jess faced and loved her deeply, and the support the children gave her was complete, unconditional and honest. She could not have asked for more. We returned home from our day at the sea content but very sunburnt, as we had not realised the strength of the sun due to the breeze. This little bit of colour made Jess look glowing and healthy again and it was hard to believe that she was facing so much.

In the days following our trip to the sea Jess developed a rash on her legs, which could have been a reaction to the seawater due to her reduced immunity. "It was a wonderful day. I had such a fun time. I don't care if I have a rash on my legs," had been Jess's answer to the doctor when we owned up to our visit to the beach. And so we laughed it off.

One of the other wishes she had made was for a picnic in the park. This was easy to organise and we invited some friends to meet us there. We split into teams playing 'rounders' for the afternoon followed by an ample and very welcome picnic. Good food and great company made the ingredients for yet another memorable day. The other items on her list were more materialistic - things she felt she wanted for her hospital stay and a new dress for her confirmation. Jess always enjoyed retail therapy when she was worried about anything, there was no doubt she was just like me in that respect. And so we made several shopping trips to find an outfit for her confirmation and other clothes that she felt she needed. I tried to fill her days with as much excitement as possible over the time leading up to her operation, I was afraid of losing my precious girl and wanted to do as much as I could for her whilst I had the chance.

Suddenly Mr de Ville de Goyet appeared in the waiting room with us, looking tired - it was now almost 8 o'clock and the operation had lasted 11 hours. He sat down and began to talk about the operation, and he was quick to inform us that she was not quite ready to come down to intensive care. He had finished his part and had left his team to stitch her up and do her dressings. He proceeded to give us the news we had waited all day to hear, and we listened intently to every word he had to say. He confirmed that the operation had been extremely difficult and that there had been a few surprises as well. The two segments of liver that Jess was left with looked completely healthy, but he had experienced difficulty in reconstructing the blood flow to these segments. They had also discovered that the tumour had grown inside the portal vein and had thus been producing cells that could have travelled around her body. He had managed to reconstruct her portal vein, a procedure that I had not thought possible, and also her bile duct had to be removed and reconstructed using a section of her bowel. The good news was that he had been able to remove the tumour, but the bad news was that it had spread. It had been found immediately attached to her diaphragm and so had spread out over the top of the liver rather than being contained wholly within it as first thought. Thus, some of her diaphragm had needed to be removed as well, which had been unexpected. He went on to say that because the tumour had spread to her blood vessels and over the top of the liver he would no longer be able to consider her for liver transplant surgery, as previously thought. We would have to wait for the histology results, which would clarify whether the tumour was made up of dead or live cells and confirm the prognosis for Jess's survival. He remained hopeful that the tumour was mostly dead cells as he said it had felt hard, but it was clear that the surgery had been very difficult and he was unsure what the outcome would be.

Mr de Ville de Goyet was holding a digital camera and he offered to show us some pictures but I declined, feeling quite queasy at the thought of it. He found this reaction quite amusing and left us with half a smile on his face. I could not help but have the utmost respect for this man. He had tried his best for Jess, that was obvious, and now we just had to hope it was enough. The news that worried me the most was that she could no longer have a transplant, which meant that if she went into liver failure following the operation there would be nothing more anyone could do. She had faced this surgery with such courage; I was going to make sure she made it through.

After our amazing consultant had left, I watched the clock constantly, this time unable to lose myself in thoughts and memories, knowing that at any minute we would see her again. Even though we would see her arrive, we had been asked to wait where we were and allow the nursing staff to get her settled at her station. Once done, someone would then come to collect us. Sure enough, just after 8.30 p.m., 11½ hours after we had said our goodbyes, the lift door opened and a trolley surrounded by a team of people hurried out and along the corridor. It was hard to see her through the activity, but I caught a glimpse - enough to know that it was her - and immediately burst into tears. The relief that finally I could see her again was enormous.

Again we waited. We were professionals by now, unable to change the path that we trod and only able to wait to be called. It was past 9 o'clock when a nurse came to collect us and we followed her down the corridor, knowing from our previous tour exactly where we were going. I went straight over to Jess and gave her a kiss, held her hand and stroked her forehead. She reacted to my presence quite clearly by squeezing my hand and groaning. She looked pale and her wispy hair which had struggled to regrow was matted with a mixture of dried blood and yellow-coloured stuff that had been used to disinfect the skin. Lots of lines linked her up to the various monitors that surrounded her and she was part-way through a blood transfusion. She was on a ventilator, as expected, but she looked peaceful, asleep, as she had been when we had last seen her. Her chest moved up and down in a falsely even way, but this did not distress me. I was relieved to be able to see that she was comfortable and just to be with her and touch her again. I was amazed that despite the sedation she seemed to know that we were with her.

I stayed by Jess's side and Jerzy disappeared to inform the family that she was doing fine. What an emotional day it had been, but at last here she was even though we still had a long way to go. After an hour or so the doctors decided to reduce her sedation to see if she would start to try to breathe for herself. We all watched her closely and, sure enough, it wasn't long before she was reaching for her tube and trying to pull it out. The decision was taken to remove it and she took her first few breaths unassisted. Every little step at this stage felt like a mountain, and we had just made it over another. With the reduction of the sedation she became more aware of her discomfort and she moaned and cried with the pain. I

71

remember whispering in her ear that the tumour was gone, the one piece of news I knew she would want to hear. She found talking hard, but she squeezed my hand intermittently to make sure I was there and was able to squeeze once for 'yes' and twice for 'no'. Therefore through me she could communicate to the nurses how she was feeling. By about midnight the intensive care team had been able to control Jess's pain and she had settled off to sleep, comfortable for the moment. I was encouraged to get some rest as well, as I would need all my strength the next day to help care for her. Jerzy had already gone to bed. We were both emotionally and physically drained, pleased to have Jess back but unsure about the results of the operation. I was worried about the risk of liver failure, as described by Mr de Ville de Goyet, knowing that there was nothing further that could be done. I walked off up the corridor to the parents' accommodation, my brain feeling numb following the events of the day. Unable to process any more information or even to think sensibly, I climbed into bed. I don't remember my head touching the pillow.

I was awakened suddenly by a knock at the door. "Kirsty, Jess's mum, are you there?"

I responded, although very dazed.

"Jess is asking for you."

I thanked the nurse for coming to find me and got dressed immediately. My heart was thumping. I had woken up frightened that something awful had happened. The nurse had assured me she was fine but she just wanted me there. It was almost 6.00 a.m. and I had slept for about 5½ hours, although it felt like only a few moments. I ran along the corridor to intensive care, I wanted to be with her so much too. She saw me enter the room and was clearly delighted although in extreme discomfort. She couldn't remember anything of the night before, but had realised I was not there when she woke up that morning and had asked for me. The nurses told her all about the operation and how we had been with her when she came out of theatre, and she was amazed that she couldn't remember. She looked completely different to me now - so much better than the night before. She was wide awake and aware of her surroundings, and although it was painful to move she was comfortable. The bed had been set at an angle to help and she was coming to terms with the various lines that were attached to her. She had one in her neck that felt quite awkward, but the play specialist had warned her about it on the day before the operation by using a teddy to which all the same lines had been attached. She had a tube up one nostril, which went down to her stomach, an oxygen tube attached to the other nostril, and a drain the size of a garden hosepipe that went directly into her side. This drain made me feel quite ill when I first saw it. Jess's bed had been brought down from the ward with the intention of transferring her onto it before we left intensive care. Once she was comfortable she could then return to the ward. It took about eight people to move her. She was in a lot of pain and everything seemed to hurt, and I am sure the fear of being moved didn't help either. However, once on the bed she looked much more comfortable, and she soon settled into the cool clean sheets and fell asleep. She slept then for much of the day, unaware of being transferred back to the ward. There were so many machines and drips surrounding her bed that it was hard to fit a chair into her bed space. I elected to stand for much of the day, and as her bed was very high I could comfortably hold her hand. I watched her sleep, content just to be there after the trauma of the previous day. Andrew came to visit and brought his girlfriend onto the ward to meet us for the first time. She seemed lovely and I apologised for being so antisocial the day before. I think as a mother herself she understood.

Over the next few days Jess struggled to regain her mobility. It was hard work for her - she was suffering as a result of the bases of both lungs collapsing as well as with the pain from the surgery. I was constantly with her, encouraging her and physically helping her to move with the aid of the physiotherapist. They wanted her to get moving quickly, but it was hard being attached to so many things. As each line was removed one by one so it became easier. The breathing exercises helped enormously and by the third day she was clearly doing very well. Her blood results had returned to normal and she was slowly and steadily making good progress.

Over the ten days that she spent recovering she showed outstanding courage, still finding room to think about other children on the ward. We gave her some helium balloons to decorate her bed, which she gave to some of the younger children before she left. One little girl had been diagnosed with non-Hodgkin's lymphoma and was very ill indeed. Jess didn't manage to speak to her, but her mum came over and found some strength in talking to Jess about her treatment. Sadly this little girl died following her biopsy; she was so ill I don't think she ever regained consciousness. This was something that affected everyone on the ward and reminded me how close we had come to the same outcome, although I never mentioned that to Jess. I wrote a card to this little girl's mum, giving our contact details, which the ward staff passed on, although I never heard from her again. Jess got stronger and stronger and was eventually able to walk a few steps, gradually increasing that to a stroll down the ward and back again. The drain was the last thing that was removed, shortly before we were able to go home. This is the one and only time throughout Jess's treatment that I came close to fainting; it was truly horrible. Once the stitches were removed it was supposed to pull out, and it did, but it was so big and much longer than I had expected. I comforted Jess from the other side of the bed and I really could not watch. Not surprisingly, poor Jess got quite hysterical about it and the nurse tried to be as quick as she could, but I was so glad when it was over. It took Jess a while to get over that: the hole left by the drain took a long time to heal and leaked this horrid yellow stuff. However, Jess was remarkably constant in her courage and never complained once.

She was visited by family and friends, receiving lots of cards, presents and flowers. Jerzy marched in one day with an enormous cuddly dog, which he had walked up the road with as though he had an old friend under his arm. Jess adored this dog and it always remained a constant favourite. As Jess got stronger the teacher on the ward found her a computer to use and she also took part in various activities arranged by the play therapists. We were so excited for her. At last the tumour was gone and she was so pleased that Mr de Ville de Goyet had been able to do the operation. We were all so very hopeful. Jerzy came and went a few times due to work commitments, but he tried to bring Gemma and Stewart when he could.

Unfortunately, about a week later I was informed that the histology of the tumour was not good: the tumour was still alive despite all the months of chemotherapy Jess had endured. Although it had been removed, the consensus of opinion was that it would grow back again and when it did there would be very little that could be done. I listened to this but did not tell Jess as she needed to recover, so as far as she was concerned she was on the up. How could I tell her that now?

Eventually the day came when Jess was discharged from Birmingham Children's Hospital. How elated we all felt that against all the odds Jess had survived, and we rejoiced in being able to bring her home.

She went from strength to strength and three weeks later, when visiting Mr de Ville de Goyet at his outpatient clinic, it was confirmed that Jess was well enough to be given her last dose of chemotherapy. At the same time he reiterated to her that he would not be able to do a liver transplant because the tumour would grow again in the new liver. We understood his reasoning and we realised that we just had to hope that by some chance it would not grow again. Jess was fully aware of the situation by this stage. She knew the tumour had remained alive even after the strongest chemotherapy regime she could have been given and she now knew that she could not have a liver transplant. She knew everything but she had not put it all together and worked out how volatile her situation was.

Jess was happy to be getting some strength back and she had started to go to school again. She so wanted to do well in her SATs. With some encouragement from her home tutor and lots of help from her headmaster, Jess sat all her SATs without taking the extra time allocation to which she would have been entitled. She wanted to take them on a par with everyone else and felt it would be unfair on the others if she took extra time. She gained level 4s and 5s in all of her exams, a truly outstanding result considering the battle she had personally fought for the whole of that school year.

Jess's final chemotherapy was a real struggle. Although the dose was reduced due to the size of her remaining liver, she felt very unwell and got terribly depressed. I stayed with her, as always. I read to her and remained by her side, although she did not want to talk or do anything. Then suddenly, out of the blue, Jess said, "I want to go home. I don't want any more chemo." There had been a slight spillage of her medicine, which had upset her greatly, and she had not been able to settle back into it again. However, a nurse came to talk to Jess and, although she was very down, he managed to persuade her to continue with the treatment for the moment. She fell asleep, not wanting to speak to anyone.

Afterwards I went up the corridor with the intention of making a cup of tea, feeling really sad and unsure about what the future held. The nurse caught up with me and invited me to sit a while and talk with him. The conversation that followed was not what I had been expecting at all. I asked him what was going to happen next, as Mr de Ville de Goyet had said that Jess needed to have either further chemotherapy or radiotherapy in order to try to arrest the disease. As far as I was aware, there was not going to be any further treatment and nobody was talking to me about it. He started to look tearful, which surprised me, and then he said, "Are you ready to hear that Jess might only tick on for another six months?" He explained to me that it was generally felt that Jess would relapse fairly quickly. The course of treatment she had been given should have done the trick, but it hadn't, and there wasn't anything else we could do but wait and see. We sat and talked for a while longer and I remember crying a lot. He arranged for us to get together with Nicky in the afternoon, as he felt the time had come for us all to sit down and discuss the options together.

After lunch Nicky joined us and we sat and talked it all through. Apparently Jess's body had not handled the chemotherapy very well. It had knocked her bone marrow back fairly substantially and her kidneys had also struggled to cope. In Nicky's opinion the chemotherapy she was having at that time was doing no more than holding things for a while. Her body would not be able to cope with constant chemo as the drugs were too strong, and if she did continue she would end up dying from the effects of the treatment rather than the cancer. They were investigating radiotherapy as an option, but it looked unlikely that she would be able to tolerate this either: as she did not have very much liver left the rays would be likely to affect her stomach and cause her to be very ill, and they were also concerned again about liver failure. In short, it wasn't looking good and, although no timescale could be put on it, the tumour was likely to return very quickly. We would then have to think very carefully about quality of life and control of the symptoms rather than a cure. Nicky was crying at this point as well. She was gentle in the way she spoke and as a mother herself she knew how devastating this news was to me and she felt our pain. Nicky never put up any barriers and always explained things just as they were. She knew that Jess hated to be in hospital and we talked about keeping her out of pain so that she could remain at home to die. In her lowest moments of treatment, Jess had wanted to talk about dying and I knew she would not want to be in hospital. I felt completely shattered. After all we had been through, Jess had survived this massive operation and all her treatment. She had no visible signs that she was still suffering from cancer and yet I was being told she might not survive for very much longer. This was really devastatingly hard news to digest and I struggled to take it all on board.

Jess finished her treatment and we returned home. In the days that followed I sat Jess down and told her what had been said. I told her that things did not look good but also that I remained hopeful and I wanted her to as well. We had been through far too much to give up now and if hope was all we had then we had to cling on to it.

We had an appointment to see her consultant in Bristol and knew that we would have a better idea about radiotherapy at that point. We returned from that appointment a little bit more hopeful, as the consultant had confirmed that she had known other children in Jess's situation who had surprised everybody. I think she was trying to help us to realise that there was always hope. We were told that no radiotherapy treatment would be undertaken at the moment, as they wanted to wait and see. Although there were other chemo drugs, she currently had no tumours to measure and so we would have no idea whether the treatment was working or not. The advice was to make the most of our time and enjoy the summer holidays. Jess was looking forward to starting her new school and we just had to get on with living. They would look at possible treatments if and when the cancer returned, and the longer she went without relapsing would be a good sign.

Jess was afraid and following these conversations with Nicky and her consultant in Bristol she felt the need to talk about dying. She seemed to see that as being her future. I encouraged her to believe in herself, to carry the love and hope we had with her always; she had to believe she could get better. I explained it to her using the horse-racing game that we often played as a family: "Occasionally an outsider comes home first and that's what you have to cling on to." She understood. The chances weren't good, but while there was a chance then there was still hope. We put these discussions behind us and concentrated on life, getting back to being a family.

I found the easiest way to continue was to believe that everyone was wrong. Looking back, this was a cynical approach but it worked well for me at the time. We don't choose to behave as we do in these situations, it's almost as though instinct takes over. To believe that the professionals had got it wrong meant that Jess had a better chance and this made life easier. Jess looked so much better, she was able to enjoy herself and play with her friends and, above all, she was looking forward to her new school.

We engaged in buying a new school uniform and books, she thrived on the warmer weather and her hair noticeably started to grow back. She was clearly feeling hugely better spiritually, emotionally and physically. Starting the forthcoming term at her new secondary school (Courtfields Community School in Wellington) seemed to be the focal point for all this new-found positive energy. The thought of rejoining her school friends at the beginning of this new journey for them all was immensely important to her. She finally had the opportunity of leaving her treatment behind: a treatment she dismissed as a bad memory, another lifetime that was not now. She really reached for her future full of courage and committed to making the most of every opportunity that might come her way.

Chapter 8

It was now July 2001, and plans were made to have Jessica's Hickman line removed. She had hated it and couldn't wait to be rid of it. She so loved the water and it had placed so many restrictions on her enjoyment of swimming. It was not easy to arrange to have it removed as priority was always given to children who needed to have them inserted so that treatment could start, and rightly so. I remembered how anxious we had felt when commencing the treatment. Now Jess had finished and we therefore had to wait for the opportunity to come up. Our impatience was brought on by an impending family holiday in Wales, which she was really looking forward to, and if her line could be removed in time for that it would mean so much to her. I offered to find the money for it to be removed privately, even though we couldn't really afford it, as I knew how much it meant to her. Sadly she had to come to terms with the fact that it would not be removed until September, shortly after starting her new school.

Throughout the final stages of Jess's treatment and her operation I had spoken on a number of occasions to the deputy head of Courtfields Community School. She was full of kindness and understanding, wanting to do all she could to help Jess make the transition. Coming from a tiny village school, Courtfields was a daunting prospect, as it was for most youngsters leaping from the safety of their primary education, but Jess had other concerns in the back of her mind. Most children worry about how they look and about fitting in or finding their way around, and Jess worried greatly about her appearance. Steroids had formed part of her treatment and these had added to her solid build, and she still had very little hair which she desperately encouraged to grow. She worried that others might not accept her changed appearance, and wondered if she would fit in and be able to be as happy as she desperately wanted to be. It had been such a long time since she had attended school on a full-time basis, so she also worried about the work, keeping up and whether she would have the energy to complete all that was asked of her.

The two induction days for Courtfields approached and Jess had long set her heart on attending both days. She wanted to start her time at this school not showing anyone her weakness. She didn't want any special concessions, she didn't want any pity, she just wanted to be one of a crowd. I worried about her stamina and if she would be able to cope. She had not fully recovered from her surgery and still found walking any distance hard work. Here she would have to be up and down staircases, keeping up with her friends, and she wanted to hide her fears. The deputy head, Mrs Gibson, made sure that all Jess's lessons were on the ground floor and a mentor was assigned to her to look out for her and help with any difficulties. Through one of the cancer charities we had been offered a family break that week, but Jess had been so determined to go to the induction days that we cancelled the trip so that she could join in with everyone else.

I so admired her strength of character, courage and sheer determination; nothing was going to stop Jess from achieving her aim. She completed both days with style and thoroughly enjoyed every minute. She wore a scarf on her head to disguise her lack of hair and I know some of the boys decided to make fun of her, but by all accounts she stuck up for herself. She slept for about three days afterwards but the experience gave her the confidence to look forward to September and the thought of returning to school filled her with pride.

With these important two days behind us we set about enjoying the remainder of the summer break. We bought a ten-foot circular trampoline as a birthday surprise for Gemma and Stewart, knowing that the gentle exercise would be great for Jess too. It was wonderful to see her bouncing up and down, and she loved it. I'm sure she felt a sense of freedom as she flew through the air and I remember how she laughed. Our neighbours were an elderly couple and they have often reminisced about holding a conversation with her over the six-foot garden fence as she appeared intermittently over the top of it! I clearly remember looking back at the house from across the road and seeing Jess appearing above the garden shed, and each time she appeared she would make a funny face or position her arms and legs differently to make me laugh. She did make me laugh; it was fantastic to see the old carefree Jess shining through. We rejoiced in her happiness and loved every minute of the time we shared together.

Jess was doing so well that we decided the time had come for us to think about moving house. We had put it off due to her treatment, but we had struggled for enough living space since Jerzy had joined us and we recognised that it had to be done. His flat in London was snapped up quickly and was sold subject to contract, so this put us in the position of being able to put in an offer if we found a house that was suitable. We hoped to be able to buy before selling my house, in order to make the process a bit more straightforward. Knowing we did not have to complete on both properties on the same day appealed to me greatly. We were due to go on holiday for the first two weeks in August and therefore, in between enjoying quality time with the children, we set about trying to find a new home for us all. The children were excited about looking for a house and this process also helped us all to look to the future. For the first time in ages we were making plans again.

The first week in August proved to be a week never to be forgotten. Apart from packing to go away on the 4th, we arranged to view a couple of houses on an estate in Wellington, within walking distance of Courtfields. We were warned that a couple of offers had been made on one of them but nothing had been formally agreed as neither party had received a firm offer on their own properties. When we visited the first house we found that it was everything we wanted: spacious, four bedrooms, a huge kitchen and a conservatory. It even had a utility room, which I was particularly excited about. It felt welcoming and I remember experiencing the overwhelming feeling that I could take care of Jess there. Before we said our goodbyes the children had all decided who was having which room as though we had already agreed to buy. The next house felt gloomy by comparison and, although very similar, it didn't capture us all in the same way that number 84 had. We drove straight home and put in an offer for the full asking price, and as Jerzy's sale in London was due to complete in only a few weeks the offer was accepted. We only had a few days to put the wheels in motion before we were off to Wales. It was all a bit of a rush but at the same time it was so exciting. We had found our new home, a new start for us all.

That same night we were visited by some representatives from the Make-A-Wish Foundation, a charity that grants wishes for children with life-threatening illnesses. Although we had chosen to believe that Jess was going to survive, the fact remained that she still qualified for a wish because officially she had a very poor prognosis. They arrived bearing gifts for her brother and sister so they would not feel left out in any way. Jess was given the opportunity to talk about her four favourite ideas for wishes: Disney World; swimming with dolphins; meeting Hear'Say; and a pair of roller boots. She was asked to put them in order of preference, and I think she thought she was going to get all four wishes and so she put the roller boots first. However, her favourite wish was to go to Disney World. She wanted us all to have a special Christmas together after the sadness of the year before. We had to wait to see if the wish was approved, but just the thought of it was enough to fill Jess with tremendous excitement.

Earlier in the year I had tried to arrange a trip to Disneyland in Paris, but I had been unable to organise any insurance. The window between treatments was not big enough to allow further investigation and therefore we'd had to abandon the idea. The company I worked for had had a whip round and gave us a substantial donation towards the cost, so we used this money to pay for the second week of our holiday in Wales instead. Jess was so happy that she might have the opportunity to go to Florida, and she found it hard to find the patience to wait and see if it was approved. So, in one day we had found a home and the opportunity of a possible trip to Florida on the horizon for Jess. We were all carried on her wave of excitement with her.

The day before we left for Wales an estate agent called round to value my house with a view to putting it on the market once we returned. There was no hurry to sell, but I thought we might as well start things moving. Saturday 4 August 2001 arrived and we loaded up the car with three children, Jerzy, myself and Jet, along with a vast amount of luggage and set off on the long drive to North Wales for the first week of our holiday. We were content in the knowledge that we had put the wheels in motion to buy our new home, had organised to sell mine and had met with the Make-A-Wish Foundation. Jess seemed really well, Gemma and Stewart were in good spirits, and it all felt wonderful.

Because we did not know if Jess would be on continued treatment we had been late booking our holiday and had been unable to get two consecutive weeks in the same place. Therefore, we'd had to book two separate weeks, the first in North Wales and the following week in South Wales. It seemed like a real adventure going to two separate places and it was just as well because the first campsite we stayed at was not that brilliant. However, we were in good spirits and made the best of it despite the bad weather. The beach and the scenery were spectacular and we enjoyed many walks along the grassy sand dunes with Jet. Jess's stamina was building up and her hair had grown considerably. Despite the fluctuating weather of this first week she soon developed a healthy glow along with Gemma and Stewart. We had managed to get hold of some special dressings, rather like cellophane, which meant that we could wind Jess's line up and cover it completely so that she could go swimming. I really wish we had known how to do this before, as Jess was far less restricted in her activities and rejoiced in being able to swim again. Her immunity seemed to have recovered and we were less concerned about possible infection. How good it felt to be away from home together. We were just an average family on holiday with no worries and everything to hope for and look forward to. During that first week we had begun to relax and, although not completely at one with our surroundings, we looked forward to our 'second holiday' in South Wales.

The second week was much better: the campsite was wonderful and the accommodation fantastic. Jess immediately had to check out the swimming pool, which, just like the rest of the site, was spotlessly clean and well maintained. There was a fun water chute there and, although I took some persuasion to join in, I soon found I enjoyed it immensely. For a change the children had to keep up with me! My best memory of Jess there will always be the dance machine. She had discovered these new machines in North Wales but by the time we ventured south she had mastered the technique. They were a cross between 'Simon Says' and a jukebox, and you had to stand in the middle of a small platform divided into nine squares and would be instructed by lights to step onto the other squares in a particular dance sequence in time to the music. Jess became very professional at this and spent much of her allowance on furthering her skill. She really did look good when she was dancing, and around the machine would be other girls copying her movements in the hope of getting better themselves. From behind it looked quite wonderful to see a crowd of people all spontaneously making the same stepping movements. In her own way she was quite proud of her success, but at £2 a go this new-found passion soon ate into her pocket money.

South Wales also brought a change in the weather. Although wet and breezy at times, we did have some fantastic days when it was really quite hot. We spent these precious days on the beach, which was beautiful and sandy. The huge crashing waves were tremendous fun. Jess and Jerzy spent as much time as possible playing in the waves as they rolled and tumbled onto the sand. Gemma tried to keep up but the waves kept sweeping her legs away as she wasn't quite strong enough. Jerzy and I tried to help her, but she was very determined to do it herself and didn't seem concerned when she lost her footing and ended up being washed up like a spinning bundle of bones onto the beach. Each time this happened she would spring to her feet and begin again with more determination. How happy Jess was, and she had such an infectious laugh. She rediscovered a sense of freedom there and it was wonderful to see. She laughed and played, jumping the waves and screaming in excited anticipation of the next huge surge of water to come along.

One afternoon, however, Jess suddenly found herself in a lot of pain. I'm not sure if it was the pounding water on her body and perhaps she had overdone things a little, but I obviously worried that something else was going on. She sat on the beach under a towel and cried. I wanted to take her back to the caravan but she didn't feel she could walk that far. She sat with her knees clenched up to her tummy and I found it hard to believe that moments earlier she had been having such fun.

The lifeguard station was not very far away and so I walked

over and asked if he could run Jess and myself back to the caravan in his Landrover. I explained her story briefly and he was more than willing to help, and so she was saved from the walk back. Once she had rested on the bed for a while she seemed to feel a little better. I telephoned the Children's Unit in Taunton for some advice and was encouraged not to worry. As a family we had travelled a long road with Jess and knowing that she might relapse at any time was very hard to live with. We wanted to enjoy every single minute together and we tried to forget our journey. But every time there was an episode when Jess was in pain I felt that pain too; when she cried I cried too. I knew that if the cancer was to return then it had to be found early, and then perhaps by some miracle there would be something they could do. After this episode on the beach we continued with the holiday and I buried my fear from sight, although my soul was in turmoil. I was trying not to believe that the cancer could return but at the same time I was watching for any signs, knowing that, for Jess's sake, early diagnosis would be imperative.

A couple of days later we returned from our trip, feeling refreshed and ready to face the world again. With the summer holidays almost over and the children ready to start school again, I decided the time had come to go back to work. This was hard for me after spending so much time at home with the children, but I also felt Jess had come such a long way and she wanted to rejoin her friends and establish her own life again. This meant letting go a little and giving her the chance to fly. She was so anxious to make a good, solid start at her new school and I felt the best way to help her was just to let her go.

I found my long hours difficult; it was extremely hard to concentrate when my mind had been occupied with so many other things for such a long time. I had stopped working to care for Jess in November 2000 and it was now September 2001. However, it had been made clear to me that my job would be safe. I had seen many families with dreadful financial worries on top of having to care for a child with cancer or leukaemia. I explained that I might need to have more time off if Jess relapsed and my manager continued to be very understanding. With Jess feeling so well it was good to try to get back to being normal again. Normal for us meant me working, and although a difficult change for me on some levels it actually felt good to return.

With Jerzy being back at work as well, my mum resumed picking up the children from school, which was more complicated this time as Jess was at her new school and her brother and sister were still at Nynehead. We had still not been given a completion date on the new house, but it would be so much easier once we were in Wellington as Jess would be able to cycle or walk to school and I had promised she could have her own front door key. She was very excited at the thought of all this added freedom and openly planned who she would invite to come home with her. I made her promise no parties! Once or twice when the children were with Andrew, Jerzy and I had toyed with the idea of buying all three of them new bikes for Christmas. We had looked in several shops, making comparisons on the many prices and styles, and knew that Jess really wanted a trendy new bike to get her to school. I remember driving the car down the route she would have to take to show her the way, and she was so looking forward to the freedom our new home was going to give her.

Gemma and Stewart settled back to school quickly and Jess launched herself into her new-found circle of friends. She was very positive, encouraged by her own progress and strengths, and she did so well. She was quick to learn and intelligent, she worked hard and she would often stay late in order to finish her assignments. I remember being extremely proud of her conscientious nature, although sometimes she would find it hard to keep up and to finish things in the way she wanted. Occasionally she would cry if she didn't quite understand and we tried to help her where we could. I put this down to tiredness and her naturally ambitious nature. During this time she would often talk about growing up and what she would like to do with her life. She loved children and wanted to teach. She was kind, loving and sincere; I felt she taught so much to so many without even trying. She always saw the best in people and was always prepared to give the benefit of the doubt and to help a stranger or to guide a friend. She would often receive telephone calls from friends needing help, guidance and someone to talk to. She was a guiding star and yet inwardly she carried her own fears. However, she never complained and seldom spoke to me about her own worries at this time.

As the first half of term continued, Jess worked hard but I began to be aware of changes. There were definite episodes of pain and she would be immensely tired, often feeling sick and accompanied by a thumping headache. None of her check-ups ever showed any change and her scans were clear. I was encouraged not to worry. Perhaps I had lost sight of what normal was. I was so worried that she would fall ill again that I'm sure I was perceived as making a fuss. As half-term approached Jess became worse. She found it hard to jump on the trampoline for very long, getting out of breath very quickly. She once said to Jerzy, "See, I can't even do that anymore," becoming angry and upset. Not surprisingly, I began to worry immensely and this affected my ability to work. I spoke on the telephone often to the hospital, convinced that something was wrong and that it was being missed. I suppose this time held echoes of the past; a time remembered when I knew something was wrong and allowed myself to be reassured. I had come to regret being so passive and inwardly I felt this time I had to behave differently. Eventually an ultrasound scan was arranged, to appease my worries more than agree that there was a problem. We waited anxiously for the results of the scan, which again concluded that nothing was wrong. It was hoped that the reassurance this result would give us and the rest that Jess would get from the half-term break would make everything good again. I even started to feel as though I had lost sight of my own judgement. Even though Jess did not seem at all well, everyone was telling me that she was fine.

Feeling helpless, alone and not believed, I decided to wait and watch Jess closely. I felt I was being perceived as a paranoid mum who had lost all sense of rational thought. I was told this was 'understandable after all we had been through'. I could do nothing more than to stand back for the moment. This was an extremely difficult time for me, as I knew that if Jess were to relapse an early diagnosis would be vital. There might be further treatment that could be tried: different drugs and maybe even radiotherapy. I felt as if no one was listening even though I could see distinct changes in Jess's abilities and progress. She was having clear episodes of pain and despite her previous determination to put it all behind her and reach for her future even she was feeling as though the cancer had returned.

I was trying to continue working, at the same time caring for Jess's needs and also looking after Jerzy, Gemma and Stewart. My fears for Jess's future became all-consuming and the fact that no one heard me despite my frenzied phone calls made me question my own sanity. I decided to seek help and started having counselling via the Rainbow Centre in Bristol. This gave me an opportunity to talk openly about my fears and to explore my feelings. My counsellor, a very composed and calm lady, was incredibly helpful and listened to me with both compassion and understanding. Her visits did not take the fear away but helped me put order in my life again; she gave me back my strength and my ability to fight. Thus we continued from day to day, not really knowing what was happening but just keeping going and trying to look forward to our impending move. A new start in a new house: perhaps life would improve after all?

Chapter 9

The beginning of November brought with it the prospect of fireworks. Great excitement came over the children at the thought of another bonfire night. The 5th of November had been ideal weather: a cool crisp day, clear skies and very dry, although the ground was slightly damp underfoot. There was that definite bite of winter in the air as we set off in anticipation of a family evening together. I made sure that the children were all wrapped up warm and we drove to a local scouting event in Taunton. We had to park a short walk away but Jess felt strong and so we set off, following the crowds of people who were surging along the road in the same direction. It was a popular event and we had to queue to get in. The crowds of families stood around talking amongst themselves, their words creating a freezing mist as they met with the bite of the evening air.

Once inside we found various stalls dotted around the large, gently slopping field: a coconut shy, a hot-dog stand, some boat swings and a stall selling general bric-a-brac. We amused ourselves by wandering around these stalls while we waited for the lighting of the bonfire. Stewart loved having a go on a coconut shy; he had managed to win a couple of times in the summer and often tried his luck whenever presented with the opportunity. He was a happy, unwavering little chap and we all marvelled at his determination, but unfortunately tonight was not his night, although he was very gracious in his disappointment.

We moved on and after purchasing a hot dog each we took our place in the crowd as near to the bonfire as possible in order to admire the imminent firework display. As we watched the jets of exploding colour stretch across the sky I remembered years gone by; occasions when I had witnessed the children, in the same way as this night, marvelling at the wonder of a similar spectacle. The showers of light darting this way and that were accompanied by their familiar noises: huge bangs and hissing sprays of colour, loud but comforting at the same time. I remembered in particular New Year's Eve 1999, the new millennium, when we had spent the evening with Steve and Sarah. I closed my eyes and remembered how all the children had delighted in the excitement of that night. Midnight had brought the onset of firework displays. We had let off our own fireworks but then stood and watched in wonder as the night sky, as far as we could see, was lit with fantastic colours. Jess had been moved to tears at this sight, so unexpected and so beautiful. The bells of all the local churches filled the night air with their music and we all delighted in the hope, love and excitement the new millennium might bring.

The bonfire was raging and projecting a welcome warmth across the crowd as the fireworks drew to a close. Gemma and Stewart began to run around, chasing one another as the crowd began to disperse. We stayed where we were for a moment, not wanting to get caught up in the rush, and Jess began to join in with the other two, laughing and giggling as she always did and carefree for a moment. Then suddenly, completely out of the blue, Jess fell to the ground in pain. Screaming and bent double in her sudden agony, she lay on the damp ground - such a contrast from just moments before. I ran to her and held her tight. Luckily we were still very close to the fire and its warmth rained down on us, helping her to sit still and let the pain pass. As the car suddenly seemed a very long way away, Jerzy took Gemma and Stewart and walked on in the hope that he could bring it closer. I remained with Jess for some good while on the ground, cuddled up in the light of the bonfire. Tears ran down our faces and, although I tried to comfort her, we both knew that there was definitely something very wrong. I looked down at her face: her eyes were closed as she cuddled into me but the warmth of the fire reflected on her smooth skin and streams of tears glistened down her cheeks.

Despite the crowds of people no one noticed our despair and soon we were amongst only a handful of people remaining in the field. Jess had regained some strength at this point and the pain had passed, so we decided to start walking back in the hope that Jerzy would meet us halfway. Jess was very quiet and I can only guess how she was feeling as she couldn't speak about it. I felt her sadness; she was frightened and angry. I promised that I would speak to the hospital in the morning. Surely they would listen to me now?

We made our way home. The evening had started so well, but we had returned disappointed and unsure about Jess's plight. It was late and I encouraged the children to go straight to bed when we got in. Jess was tearful and found it hard to sleep, so I stayed by her side and stroked her forehead. As a baby Jess had been easily comforted in the same way. She had so often fallen asleep in my arms and I would creep away once I knew she was settled. When she was a little older she would joke with me by pretending to be asleep and then laugh just when I thought it was safe to retire. Throughout her treatment I had similarly knelt on the floor beside her bed. Sometimes I would find myself in this position for hours and often I would fall asleep with my head laid on the pillow next to hers. She found strength in this closeness and often called out to be near me. Tonight she wanted me to say it was all going to be fine, but I couldn't. All I could do was promise to speak to the hospital and try to arrange a scan as soon as possible. Eventually she drifted to sleep and I crept downstairs to Jerzy, and we spent an anxious evening deciding what to do for the best.

First thing in the morning I telephoned the hospital and explained the events of the previous evening, which seemed to spark an element of concern in the medical team. I felt that I had been heard this time and another scan was scheduled for the following Friday. This was the day we were due to exchange contracts on our new house and Jerzy had already kept the day clear for this reason. He persuaded me to continue to go to work that week, as I was in the middle of a training course, and he would take Jess to the hospital on that day. It felt strange letting Jerzy take control like this, as usually I accompanied Jess to these appointments. However, in one way I was glad he was going because I was feeling as though I had made a nuisance of myself. And so for those few days until her appointment the children continued to go to school as normal, I went to work and Jess stayed home with either my mum or Jerzy. We desperately tried to look forward to our impending move and I took out my frustrations on packing.

Friday came all too soon and I went off to work as usual, although understandably anxious about Jess's scan. She felt more confident on that day; the pain had gone and the memory of our firework night had faded a little. I made them promise to let me know as soon as the results were confirmed to them. My day was a strange one. I couldn't concentrate or apply myself in any way and I began to realise that I would have been better off going to the hospital after all, but I also knew that Jess would be fine with Jerzy. The hours ticked by and still no news, and it was not until about 3.00 p.m. that finally I was informed Jess was on the phone. I immediately took the call, anxious to know that all was fine - but it wasn't.

I could hear the tears in Jess's voice as she said, "Mummy?"

She paused, and I encouraged her to tell me how it had gone.

"It's back, the cancer's back, mummy, and I've got four tumours."

Her voice trailed off into floods of tears and she handed the phone over to Jerzy, who confirmed more details to me. I didn't take much in as complete shock took over. Although I had half expected bad news, I had tried to believe that everything would be okay. I asked to speak to Jess again and I told her that I would be home in only a few minutes and that I loved her, and tried my best to reassure her.

I made my apologies and left immediately. I was shaking and crying; I felt sick to my stomach that I had been proved right. How I drove home I have no idea. The journey only took about ten minutes but each minute seemed like an hour. I wanted to hold Jess in my arms; I wanted to take it all away from her, but of course I couldn't. She trusted in my courage and she needed me to be strong; to fight for her and to support her. She already knew I would never give up hope. Sure enough when I eventually made it home she was waiting for me by the door just as she had right back in the beginning. She ran out to greet me, her eyes full of tears and the pain of this dreadful news. We went in and sat together on the sofa, where she cuddled into me and drifted off to sleep, exhausted from the many emotions she had flying around in her head. Jerzy took the opportunity to fill me in on the details of the day. The CT scan had indeed identified four small tumours spread around her remaining liver. A further ultrasound scan had been arranged, as it had been only two weeks since the all-clear had been given. This scan confirmed the presence of the same four tumours and the conclusion was drawn that these growths had appeared quickly over this short time, a measure of the aggressive nature of the disease. Nicky had sat Jerzy and Jess down in one of the consulting rooms to give them the bad news and she has often remarked on Jess's reaction. She didn't think about herself; instead her first response had been to say, "How are we going to tell Mum?"

We already had an appointment booked for the following Monday with Jess's consultant from Bristol, who held a clinic every month in Taunton. Our last meeting had been more positive as at that time Jess was doing really well and there were no visible signs that her problems had returned. Now my fears had been proved right, options for treatment would be discussed at this next appointment. We would therefore have to get through the weekend and face Monday when it came. Gemma and Stewart came home from school and all weekend we tried hard to distract Jess from her fears and to be as positive as we could. This was not difficult as we had successfully exchanged contracts on the new house and completion was set for the following Friday. What a week this was turning into. The children excitedly helped to pack up their things and the anticipation of the move took over all of us. It was good to plan for our future and it helped that all the children were very happy indeed with our choice of new home.

Not being entirely sure what the outcome of Jess's appointment on Monday would be and knowing how we had been sent to Bristol Children's Hospital before, I decided to try to get as far ahead of myself as I possibly could during that weekend. The children were enthusiastic about being involved and this excited energy meant I could concentrate on getting much of the house cleared. I got ahead with the washing and ironing and made sure that Gemma and Stewart's school things were easy to find in case Jess and I had to go away and Jerzy was left to cope on his own again. This was not a thought I relished, but my experience thus far had taught me to be as organised as possible. Not only were we facing being separated by Jess's treatment again, but also our move was hanging over our heads like a real obstacle to climb. The new start we had allowed ourselves to look forward to had now come right at the wrong time, and as anyone knows moving house can be stressful at the best of times. By Monday, however, we were as organised as we could be and, with Gemma and Stewart at school, Jerzy, Jess and I headed to the hospital.

We sat pensively and waited our turn in the children's outpatient waiting room. We had done this so many times before, but today felt different. We were all overwhelmed and consumed in thought. How could Jess have come through so much and still lose her fight? Jerzy and I tried so hard to remain cheerful whilst we waited, but Jess saw right through the pair of us. She was very tactile and needed to be close; she knew we felt her fear. Before long we were called in, and I felt just as I had done the very first time we had been called to speak to the consultant following Jess's initial CT scan: knowing something was wrong, but not knowing what was coming next. The conversations that followed were very soul searching but in short they confirmed the results of the scans and we talked about treatment. Jess was clearly informed that it was not thought to be possible to cure her anymore. She had had the treatment most likely to have worked and this had clearly not done the trick. The plan was to control her symptoms and to look at keeping her comfortable. This is when her plight hit her for the first time. She had always known there was a chance she would not survive, but here it was being given to her straight.

"You mean I'm going to die?"

She choked back her tears as her realisation was acknowledged and disbelief came over her. She wanted to fight; she didn't want to give up hope. In recognition of this she was offered further chemotherapy but using different drugs this time. We all hoped that this might help in some way. Jess's consultant also promised to look into radiotherapy, which Jess was particularly keen to explore, although this avenue had been turned down previously. We didn't discuss too much more. The truth of her situation had been too big to swallow and Jess was overcome with emotions. I suspect, as previously, that she had so much information flying around in her head it was hard for her to make sense of anything. I know she felt let down and angry. She had taken her treatment almost as a promise that she would one day be well again. She ran out of the room crying, heading off up the corridor away from the outpatient waiting room. Jerzy and I fled in hot pursuit, saying our goodbyes in a very brisk fashion. Just what were we supposed to say?

Jess hadn't gone far and we soon caught her up. She was very angry and didn't know what to do with herself, so I held her tight and we all cried together. I didn't know what to say or do; instinct was my closest friend, as it had been since the very beginnings of her illness. Sometimes to say nothing is very powerful, along with the physical experience of being held, and Jess seemed to respond well to this. I couldn't make the cancer go away; I couldn't tell her things would seem better in the morning or put a plaster on a cut or graze that would heal. From this point on, I could only walk next to Jess and help her to accept the changes that would come over her. I could only encourage her to stay positive and to know I would always be with her.

After this visit to hospital Jess's world filled with a good deal of anger, although wanting to continue with further treatment. Her tolerance of being in hospital for any length of time diminished. She often wore her favourite T-shirt which seemed so graphically to capture her sense of self. It read 'I love my attitude problem', reflecting her knowledge that at times she grew short with people, but wearing this statement so proudly enabled her to hide her anger with the use of humour. She put up barriers aimed at certain people and she found it hard to remain her cheerful, happy self, the Jess we all knew so well. Her defence mechanisms had started to kick in. It was hard to hear her being rude or spiteful, but it was so understandable that she might react like this when considering the disappointment of her world. She was angry, and rightly so. Realistically, it was anger at her situation and it was no one's fault. In that single appointment the future she had prayed so hard for was so cruelly snatched away. Her consultant from Bristol never saw her again. Jess didn't want to see her as she hadn't told her what she wanted to hear. Even the best of us would find it hard not to be angry with those around us when faced with such devastation and the knowledge of certain death within a short space of time. She never meant it personally. All the people that had ever been involved in her care had looked after her with complete commitment, compassion and empathy for her situation. Her attitude came from her love of life; she so wanted to be like everyone else and to know a future. It was hard for her to accept the truth as it was, and indeed I felt that she tried to deny it for a while.

Once back at home, Jess and I discussed her feelings and she made it quite clear that she desperately wanted to fight on, so I telephoned Nicky to discuss the chemotherapy. It was decided to start the treatment the very next day, meaning that Jess would finish on the Friday at the same time as we completed on the house. Jess was desperate to be the first one to put the key in the door of our new home and this is what we aimed for. The drugs were very different to the ones Jess had experienced before and they made her very ill indeed. She struggled through those few days with courage. She found it very hard to continue, as she was very sick and dizzy and she became very depressed. Despite being so ill she remained determined to open the door of our house and focused on this as though it were all that kept her going. As her Hickman line had been removed, the drugs were administered through a cannula inserted into her wrist, which became sore and added to her discomfort. With no line to use, she very quickly developed a fear of needles. This was not a problem we had experienced previously, but Jess's tolerance levels had declined and her reactions to having blood taken were very distressing not just to Jess but to those around her. She was booked into Bristol Children's Hospital for a small operation to insert a further Hickman line in order to make any forthcoming treatment more tolerable. Although a new line would make her treatment easier, her unpleasant experiences surrounding this new fear of needles would stay with her and fuelled her dislike of being in the hospital even more. It was always going to be an uphill struggle for Jess to continue.

During those few days I noticed a distinct difference in the demeanour of the nursing staff. Everyone seemed to know our fears and misery. I tried to hide how I felt, but I would often find myself in tears a little way down the corridor from Jess's room. Everyone on the ward seemed to know that things weren't looking good for Jess and there was a sense of sadness in everyone's eyes. I spent a lot of time talking to Nicky, who told me that she felt the treatment Jess was having was doing little more than holding things for a while. They considered it extremely unlikely that it would provide the cure we so desperately hoped for. The speed at which the tumours had manifested themselves was worrying and Nicky felt quite doubtful whether Jess would survive for more than a few months. Inwardly I started to doubt how appropriate this new course of treatment was, but Jess had wanted to do it and I tried to support her decisions; after all, it was she that would have to go through it all. I decided that all I could do was to be there for her. My hope was as strong as ever and I knew that Jess still had the courage to fight.

Friday came eventually and Jess got herself dressed and ready to sit in the wheelchair as the last of her chemotherapy went through her lines. She was desperate to leave and the minute she was disconnected she was pushing herself up the corridor. She was grinning cheekily, as though escaping from the ward that had held her captive as a prisoner for those last few days. She was a strong character and the ward staff clearly cared deeply for Jess, but she had no intention of hanging around for fond farewells, she was gone. Laden with all her belongings and her duvet, I chased after her and we turned out of the ward into the sloped corridor that led to the car park. As she had done so often before, she let go of the wheels and sped down the slope, laughing in defiance at her condition. She loved to do this, although dangerous, and I laughed with her. This gave her a sense of freedom. She hated to be cooped up on the ward and it was so like Jess to want to stretch her wings and fly.

Once in the car we drove directly to meet Jerzy, and Jess put the key in the door of the new home just as she had promised herself she would. The house seemed so empty, but it felt welcoming and I knew we would be happy there. Isn't it strange how some houses emanate a sense of warmth and welcoming? We wandered from room to room, making plans for where items of furniture would be placed. I couldn't imagine that it would stay quite so tidy for very long! Soon my mum turned up with Gemma and Stewart, who ran excitedly around the empty rooms. We ate fish and chips for tea at our newly delivered table and chairs and then returned to our old house for an early night. Saturday would be a very busy day: the end of a truly exhausting week.

We were up extremely early the next morning to pack up the last of our things, which didn't take long, and we were soon ready to go. The removal men arrived at 8.00 a.m. and began loading the larger items onto the lorry. Gemma and Stewart joined in where they could and Stewart enjoyed running in and out of the lorry carrying the lighter boxes, although very much under the watchful eye of one of the removal men. They obviously had lots of experience with children and helped them to stay safely busy. Jess, however, was feeling extremely ill. The excitement of the day had woken her early, but she could do little more than rest on the sofa with a bowl on her lap. Despite the strong anti-emetic medication we had brought home with her, she was still feeling very sick and I felt so sorry for her. She could have gone across the road to my mum's house for some peace and quiet, but she wanted to be part of this special day and could still watch and laugh even if she couldn't do anything. The removal men knew that Jess was very ill and left the sofa until the very end so that she was comfortable, but eventually even this had to go. Jerzy and the children followed the lorry in the car. It wasn't far to the new house - only about three miles - and the first item off would be the sofa for Jess. I waved to the children as the convoy rounded the corner of our street and went out of sight. I remained behind for a while with the intention of clearing up, but it wasn't long before exhaustion started to set in: a mixture of the traumatic week we had had and the events of that day. Mum persuaded me to leave the cleaning, as my house was not due to complete for some weeks and there would be plenty of time at a later day. She was right, of course, but I didn't take much persuading really - I needed a cup of tea and the kettle had gone with everyone else!

I took a last look around. It all looked so empty and it was easy to recall the day we had first moved there. I had just left my first husband and after many months of organising I had celebrated my independence and completed on this little house. We had been happy here despite Jess's illness. This house had represented freedom to me; it was mine and no one could take that away from me. Our time here had been good. I felt tearful as I drove away, but I knew we were going to be more comfortable in our new home. Jerzy had transformed us into a family of five and there was no doubt we needed extra space. He had thoughtfully won the trust of the children and I rejoiced in the joy he so gently introduced into my life. Ultimately we needed to build a home that was ours together and I knew this move, despite Jess's relapse, was going to be a great new start for us all.

As I drove to Wellington my tearfulness subsided and when I arrived at our new home a feeling of elation took over. We had done it! Complete chaos ruled everywhere you looked, but we were there. The lorry was still being unloaded and piles of boxes and debris were amassing all over the house. Barely any space remained that wasn't soon filled with something, and in amongst this mess Gemma, Stewart and the dog were darting in and out, playfully exploring. Poor Jet ran into the patio doors a couple of times and slipped in spectacular style on the unfamiliar polished floor. Despite the chaos, however, our tired bodies had been revived by the sense of achievement. We could see the end of our day in sight and it felt really good. Jess remained on the sofa, however, still feeling very ill, but she was also happy, swept along with our euphoria and so glad to be involved with it all.

Poor Jess remained sick for much longer than we had previously experienced. The new drugs had bowled her over completely and she found it hard to bounce back. I remained at home with her; I was unable to think about working now, although I feared I might lose my job. However, Jess needed me and I had promised her I would always be there, and if that meant losing my job so be it. I was not prepared to compromise; I had to be home despite the possible consequences.

For several days Jess slept a great deal, which left me plenty of time to sort out our new home, although everything fell into place quickly and it wasn't long before we were fairly well organised. The events of that week ending with the move had completely exhausted poor Jess, but she never complained. She was pleased to have been part of the move and was really glad to have her own room. Gemma and Jess had shared a room for some years, but now Jess was getting older she needed more privacy. Jess liked to have all her little things around her and didn't like her little sister interfering. She collected all kinds of things: china dolls, ornaments and many souvenirs from trips out. Jess had put together quite a collection by now and was pleased to have a room that was safe from sisterly fingers at last!

Chapter 10

Confirmation of the relapse hit Jess understandably hard and her first dose of chemotherapy had been very difficult to tolerate. She didn't want to return to school again; she felt weak and sick, unable to walk any distance without using a wheelchair. Her operation for a new Hickman line came up quickly and we were all relieved once this was done, Jess included. Her fear of needles had escalated to such an extent that monitoring her blood had become near impossible. I tried to persuade her to return to school, if only for an hour or so here and there, but she had lost confidence in herself and worried about how her new friends would perceive her. Jess had some lovely friends and I felt she needed their friendship and support. By the time she had recovered from her Hickman line operation, two weeks had passed since her first dose of chemotherapy and the side effects of the drugs were starting to become evident. When Jess had had treatment before, her hair had fallen out gradually, getting thinner and thinner until eventually she was left with a few wispy bits. This time her hair loss was rather more dramatic, perhaps a sign that her body was not so resilient and she was more vulnerable to this regime of chemotherapy than we had first thought.

Jess was lying on the sofa watching television, her head on a cushion, while I was in the kitchen cooking the tea. Suddenly she screamed. I ran to her immediately and she met me halfway in the hall. The hair that had been in contact with the cushion was still on the cushion, leaving poor Jess with half a head of hair. As she walked towards me, further clumps were falling from her head and leaving a trail on the carpet behind her. The sadness in her eyes was immeasurable; she had willed this hair to grow with every ounce of her strength. Tears welled as she ran her hand over her head and all the hair she touched separated from her scalp. Crying bitterly, she sat back down and removed the rest of it, angrily placing it in a pile on her lap; within minutes it had all gone. She was completely shocked and ran upstairs to her room as neither Gemma nor Stewart had noticed and she dreaded their reaction. Seeing Jess pull her hair out like that stands out in my memory as one of the single most heart-rending moments of our last few months together. To Jess her hair was a symbol of her return to health and her confidence in her new school, so to lose it again was completely devastating for her. The shock of losing it so quickly affected her deeply and it was some good while before she was able to look at herself in the mirror again.

I followed her upstairs in an attempt to offer some comfort and we sifted through her cupboard to find some of the hats she had relied on before. She choked back the tears in favour of her anger, barely able to speak and visibly shaken. She didn't like any of these hats anymore, and I had to agree she seemed to have grown up such a lot over the past few months and her fashion sense had changed beyond recognition. We agreed to go to town as soon as possible and try to find some hats that suited her more mature look. She found this thought comforting, although she wanted to lie quietly in her room for a while and listen to some music. I gave her a hug and left her alone, coming downstairs to have a chat with Gemma and Stewart. I warned them both that Jess had lost her hair very suddenly and they must be careful not to upset her about it. They felt really sad for her and when she did appear they both hugged her, trying to comfort her in their own way. Gemma went to give Jess a kiss, which Jess found a bit odd as she never liked to be too close, and her reaction sent all three of them into fits of laughter. It was good to see them all laughing, it was such a tonic, and it helped us all to make light of this very awkward situation.

Despite this light-hearted moment, Jess would not return to school, as she couldn't face her friends in case her changed appearance should provoke an unwanted reaction. Preferring to hide away at home, Jess opted to have visits from the home tutor once again. I know she missed her friends and it must have been painful for her, but her fears won over. It was difficult for her and it was also difficult for me to know what to do for the best, but I lived in hope that I could persuade her to pluck up the courage to spend time with her friends again.

Following Jess's relapse I contacted the Make-a-Wish Foundation again. Our trip to Florida had been postponed due

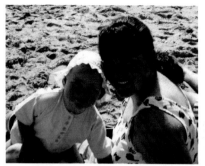

Our first day on the beach
together, Summer 1991

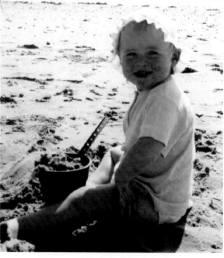

Jess proudly presents her first snowman!
February 1994

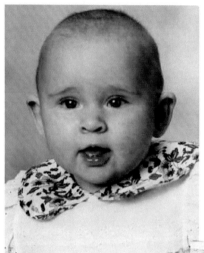

Jess 5 Months Old and sitting
up already!

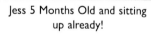

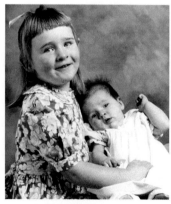

A new baby sister,
September 1993

A passion for the sand from that first day

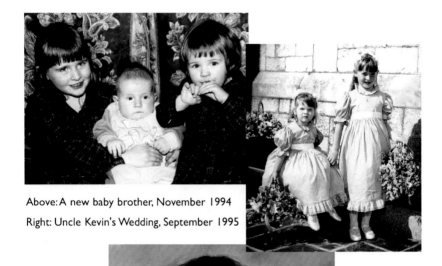

Above: A new baby brother, November 1994
Right: Uncle Kevin's Wedding, September 1995

First School
Photo,
September 1994

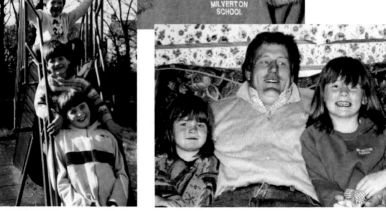

Stewart, Gemma and Jess
on a slide, September 1998

Jess & Gemma with Daddy, 1996

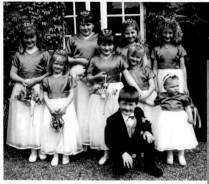

Kirsty & Jerzy's Wedding,
Left to right:
Hannah - Jess - Stasia - Katie
Ellie - Gemma - Sammy - Alice
Stewart

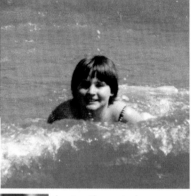

Loving the water!

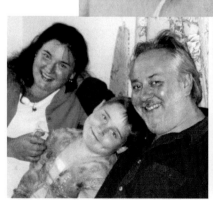

Chemotherapy was a long
battle, February 2001

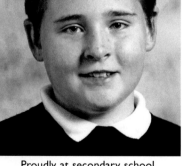

Recovering from surgery, June 2001

Proudly at secondary school,
September 2001

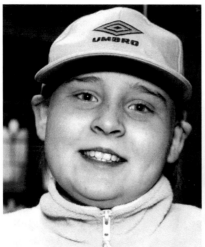

By April 2001 Jess felt much stronger

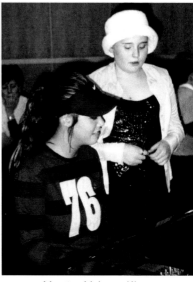

Meeting Myleene Klass.
A dream come true, November 2001

Above: Our last holiday
together in Wales,
August 2001

Right: Our last family
photo taken at
Little Bridge House,
February 2002

to the horrific attack on the World Trade Center in New York on 11 September 2001. The uncertainty surrounding further terrorist activity, particularly involving aeroplanes, had led to the Foundation's decision to cancel all trips to America until further notice. Jess had been happy to wait and see whether this decision would be reversed in the New Year, but she was well at that point and now things were very different. The Foundation agreed to arrange another wish for Jess and so planned for her to meet the band members of Hear'Say. Much of the trip was kept a secret from Jess until the last minute in case we weren't able to make it, and we nearly didn't. Jess's immunity started to wane and she became very neutropenic again, and she also needed another blood transfusion. She developed a very high temperature and had to be admitted to hospital for intravenous antibiotics over the weekend prior to her surprise trip. We were due to travel to Manchester on the Wednesday and stay there until Friday. Nicky had not expected Jess to react so dramatically to just one dose of chemo, but her previous course of treatment had damaged her bone marrow along with her kidneys and her body was obviously much less able to cope this time around. There was some positive news, however: on examination, Nicky could not feel the presence of one of the tumours quite so clearly and it was thought that there may have been a positive response to the treatment despite Jess's poor condition.

This response, however small, was very encouraging and we tried to hang on to that. Jess and I often talked about her illness but I tried to persuade her to remain positive, and I promised I would never give up hope no matter what anyone said. We tried to concentrate on willing Jess's condition to pick up in time to go to Manchester. We had learned to live for the moment and nothing else mattered to Jess at that time. As those few days went by, Jess got more and more excited, although Nicky didn't actually give her permission for Jess to make the trip until the Tuesday when, right at the last minute, her blood results showed a marked improvement. Jess was overjoyed and her euphoric celebrations lifted the spirits of everyone around her. Nicky certainly breathed a sigh of relief, as she had dreaded having to deny her consent for the trip. Jess was in a huge hurry to leave the ward and, in ritualistic style, freewheeled down the corridor, yet again defiant of the rules but celebrating not only freedom but also a dream that really was coming true!

We had quite a schedule to keep. The uncertainty as to whether we would be going on the trip or not had meant I was not as organised as I would have liked. Jerzy was unfortunately unable to join us on the trip due to work commitments, so my brother, Kevin, kindly offered to drive us to Manchester. He arrived early on the Wednesday morning in a brand new people carrier supplied by the Make-a-Wish Foundation for our use over those few days. Jess was so very happy, excited and in tremendously high spirits. It was wonderful to see her so smiley; if she had any sad thoughts on her mind she certainly didn't show it. So, together with Gemma and Stewart, we set off in eager anticipation of our unfolding adventure.

We had to stop several times on the way up to Manchester, eventually arriving at our hotel around 4.00 p.m. And what a hotel it was! It had been arranged for us to stay in five-star accommodation for two nights in one of the most expensive hotels in Manchester and Jess was treated like royalty. Kevin and Stewart shared one room and Jess, Gemma and I shared the other. The rooms were en suite and had a minibar, much to the children's delight - over the time we were there they ate all the jelly beans!

When we arrived outside the hotel the concierge unloaded the car for us and drove it away to be parked. I was glad it was a smart new car and not our dirty family car, littered with remnants of the children and their creativity. Whenever we went out we had to ask someone to fetch the car for us and it would be ready and waiting whenever we wanted it. This was a service I never quite got used to, but the whole experience of staying in such a special hotel added to our adventure and I think we all felt thoroughly spoilt. The plan of action for Jess's special wish had been left waiting for us to pick up. Jess eagerly opened the envelope, as she had not been aware of the full details until that point.

The next day, Thursday, was going to be her special day, starting with a shopping trip to Debenhams where she would have the assistance of a personal shopper to choose an outfit.

Following that we would be going to the Crown Plaza Hotel in Manchester to meet Jess's idols and then on to the Hard Rock Café for tea and to round off the day. Friday would be designated mainly to packing up and travelling home. We were given the contact details for the Make-A-Wish representatives who were due to help us travel around on the Thursday. We made contact with them but decided to have a quiet evening after our journey and meet them on the Thursday morning.

After an hour or so, Jess felt more rested and we decided to have a look around, so we took a taxi into Manchester and searched for somewhere to eat. As we wandered around we found a huge cinema that was showing the first Harry Potter film, *The Philosopher's Stone*. The children were desperate to see it, so we booked some seats and found a restaurant just opposite in which to have a bite to eat before the performance started. We had not managed to get seats in our local cinema as it was such a hugely popular film and it was easy to see why. All three of the children thoroughly enjoyed it, although Gemma and Stewart kept grabbing hold of me to hide during the scary bits. Enjoying this film together made the evening really special and a great start to Jess's adventure.

We returned to the hotel straight after the film. The children were very tired by this time, although Gemma and Jess were finding it hard to believe they were really going to meet Hear'Say and took ages getting to sleep. Jess was in a little bit of pain, mostly due to the long journey and the busy day. Once lying in bed, however, she soon started to feel better and eventually drifted off to sleep full of anticipation about the events of the following day.

Needless to say, the children were dashing around very early the next morning and we had no trouble being ready to meet our guides for the day. They were wonderful - a very special couple who cared very deeply for the children they escorted on these amazing trips. My three immediately took to them as if they were a couple of old friends and we set off, following their car en route to Debenhams. We needed to make an early start to allow Jess enough time for her shopping spree before making the short journey to the hotel where the band were staying. Her personal shopper was ready to greet her and had already gone round the store and put together some suggestions for outfits. Whilst Jess busied herself trying things on, Gemma and Stewart launched themselves into the platefuls of goodies that had been laid out for us: biscuits, crisps, yoghurts and an assortment of drinks including a welcome cup of tea.

Jess loved shopping for clothes and was very particular about her idea of fashion. For an eleven-year-old she had a very grown-up sense of how she should look and didn't really take a fancy to any of the outfits that had been suggested. Her personal shopper therefore took Gemma, Jess and myself off around the shop for a further look. This expedition proved more fruitful and we soon returned with a more promising assortment for Jess to try.

Whilst Jess was changing again, one of our guides produced a magic trick from his pocket involving a few pound coins and a little brass pot. He amused my younger two with this simple trick for ages. They were desperate to work out what happened to the coins, but they never did!

Jess emerged from the changing room looking beautiful. She had chosen a pair of black trousers with a gold tinge to them and a black and gold sparkly butterfly top. She had a white hat, which she had brought with her, and had found a matching white coat with a fur trim. She looked a picture and was clearly very pleased with the outcome. A make-up lady then appeared to give Jess a more polished look. She was so chuffed with her outfit and her final appearance was just what she had hoped for.

We gathered our things together and said our goodbyes. Jess had been given an array of presents to take away with her and was overwhelmed by the kindness she had been shown. We very graciously took our leave and made our way back to the parked cars. We had some way to travel to the hotel and not very long to do it in. The traffic seemed quite bad, but then isn't that always the way when you are in a hurry? Jess was very anxious about being late and the excitement in the car soon reached fever pitch. We arrived outside the Crown Plaza just in time and waited eagerly by the entrance to be escorted inside. Hear'Say's manager appeared along with a customer service representative for the hotel and we were shown into a huge ballroom. In the middle of this enormous room was a single grand piano with a few chairs placed around it.

What a fantastic piano it was! I had learned to play when I was very young and this was easily the finest piano I had ever played. The hotel soon admitted that they had had it delivered and tuned especially for Jess - what an honour! We tentatively made ourselves at home whilst we waited for the band members to show up. Jess was very nervous as she sat herself on a chair, unable even to look around the room and frightened to move. I sat and played a couple of tunes on the piano, unable to ignore its beauty and feeling as though it might help ease the tense atmosphere a little. Every time anyone came into the room poor Jess jumped out of her skin. She was so pleased to be there but so nervous.

Eventually Myleene Klass arrived and walked straight up to Jess, greeting her as though she knew everything about her. She hugged her and the tears ran down Jess's cheeks, and then they sat and chatted a while. She was a really lovely person and so genuinely interested in Jess. She tried to encourage her to play the piano but Jess was still too scared to move. Soon another door opened and Noel came into the room, followed shortly afterwards by Suzanne. Jess was completely overwhelmed and unable to believe that this was really happening to her. Myleene sat at the piano and played one of the group's songs. Jess joined in, singing very quietly to start with but finding confidence as the tune unfolded. When the song finished they were all crying, including Myleene. I could hardly see through the tears in my eyes; happy tears this time, understanding the joy in my little girl's heart.

Jess then sat at the piano and played 'Chopsticks'. Myleene played with her, delighting Jess so completely with her impromptu knowledge of this popular tune. This visit lasted almost an hour. All the children played and chatted with them and we were allowed to take both photographs and a video recording. Intermittently, during our time together the group sang with Jess and their manager seemed nervous about this behaviour as they were not supposed to be performing. We were so grateful that they did, however. Jess sang perfectly, nervously husky to start with but gradually gaining confidence in her surroundings. Watching her with Myleene, Noel and

Suzanne filled me with pride. I don't think they realised just how much this visit meant to Jess.

Before we said our goodbyes, Jess was invited to see them perform live at a nearby shopping centre that evening. We quickly reworked our schedule so that we could be there and planned a rest for Jess so that she could get her strength back for an hour before the evening trip. Then all three band members gave Jess a 'group hug' and, although laughing at this spontaneous behaviour, she was unable to believe the friends she had just made. Their manager seemed anxious that they should leave us now and sadly they did, but they had all left a huge impression on Jess.

We were offered a cup of tea and some drinks for the children and we sat in the foyer amongst hordes of other visitors and guests. Whilst we were relaxing, Myleene appeared again and walked up to talk to us some more. She was on her way out but kindly acknowledged us for a few minutes, which made Jess feel so important. She had behaved as though an old friend and Jess couldn't wait to tell everyone back home about her adventure - and it wasn't over yet!

After leaving the hotel we made for the Hard Rock Café to have an early tea before returning to our rooms for a brief rest and a change of clothes. Jess was glad to be able to have a lie down, as she felt a little uncomfortable and needed to stretch out. The huge scar on her tummy had remained sensitive and never completely healed properly. Jess's new trousers were a little tight and had aggravated her scar line. Behind this understandable discomfort her underlying pain was increasing even though she was taking medication, but Jess tried hard to ignore it as much as possible. Jess definitely needed this rest but was soon getting herself organised for the evening stint. Our guides returned before long and we hurried eagerly into our waiting car in order to follow them to the Trafford Centre.

This journey again seemed to take forever. It was pouring with rain and the roads were filled with crawling cars that steamed as the rain bounced off their hot shells. Excitement mounted as we arrived and made our way to the performance area, where we were all invited into a special enclosure immediately in front of the stage. Jess was assigned two female security guards to take care of her needs and they kindly made sure that she had a copy of the latest album so she could have it signed after the show. There was a lot of nervous anticipation as Jess had been asked if she would like to go onto the stage with the band in front of this huge crowd later. She definitely wanted to, but I'm not sure if the management team decided it would be too much for her as the invitation to climb the steps onto the stage never came. It didn't matter, however, and after the performance she was allowed to take the privileged first place in the queue of people waiting to file in front of the band to get the album cover signed. This was excitement enough and a chance to see her friends again and hug Myleene goodbye.

Jess was exhausted by the time we returned to the hotel, but the memories of that day filled her heart with wonder and her eyes reflected her sheer delight. She slept really well and the next day we packed up and returned home. The journey home was a quiet one, as we were all thoughtful and I guess each of the children had their own experiences replaying in their minds. My thoughts circulated around seeing Jess, happy and joyful, rejoicing in new friends and putting her difficult situation to one side for a moment. I was glad that we were able to be honest with her, so she knew everything and was able to make decisions about her care, but I often felt that she carried the weight of so much for one so young. This adventure had been about living for the moment and it felt really refreshing: a chance just to 'be'; together, happy and with no anticipation of fear.

Chapter 11

The days following our adventure in Manchester drifted by in a haze of disbelief and recovery. The children were very keen to tell anyone prepared to listen about our trip and Jess would show her video to all her visitors with extreme pride. It had certainly been the realisation of a dream. Jess was completely consumed by the new friendship she had struck up with Myleene and the other members of the band and she often asked if she could contact them again. This was a very difficult request because any suggestion of further contact had been ignored and I was well aware that their lives probably led them to meet other children just like Jess on many occasions. Knowing that our visit was unlikely to have made the same impression on the band as it had on Jess, and yet not wanting to disappoint her, I would tell her that I would try to contact them. In reality, however, I didn't feel I could approach the Make-A-Wish Foundation again after they had already done so much to help us and had arranged that marvellous trip at very short notice. The trip had left Jess wanting more, but I felt that it would have been ungrateful to ask for further help.

After a few days Jess was due to be admitted to hospital again and further developments would send the memory of our Hear'Say trip to the very back of our minds. Our trip had given us a brief chance to forget Jess's fragile situation, but we were to be brought back to reality very abruptly. Gemma and Stewart returned to school and as it was the beginning of December 2001 they became engrossed in the school preparations for Christmas, including the school play. Our previous Christmas had been a very sad affair in the wake of Jess's diagnosis and our very late and unprepared return from Bristol Children's Hospital on Christmas Eve. We had tried our best but the fact remained that Christmas 2000 had fallen understandably well short of the fun time we were all accustomed to. I was therefore determined to make this Christmas so much better, even though the phrase, "This is more than likely going to be Jess's last," would come up in conversation with various professionals.

With Gemma and Stewart back to school and the anticipation of Christmas building in their hearts, Jess and I returned to hospital for the second dose of her new regime of chemotherapy. The response to the first dose had been positive and, despite losing her hair, Jess had initially felt things were going well. On examination the biggest of the tumours appeared to have receded a little, although Jess's bone marrow had struggled to cope and her blood count had fallen through the floor, giving her an unexpected period of neutropenia. However, Jess arrived on the ward feeling positive and with her new Hickman line in place she was persistent in her desire to continue with the treatment. The first knock-back came with Nicky's initial assessment of Jess's condition before treatment started. Jess had been experiencing more pain and she was very tender on examination. The largest of the tumours (which had become a benchmark for her treatment) was more prominent again and this gave rise to the feeling that the initial response to this new regime of drugs had been short lived. Poor Jess was devastated, and her confidence and trust started to crumble. However, the new course of treatment was started and once left alone we talked a little. I sat by her bed and she cuddled up to me, soon falling asleep. In the wake of bad news this became the norm for Jess. She would cry and then shut down, sleep being her protection against awkward and unwelcome conversation.

Later that day Jess had a few visitors and as it was the first day of treatment she was feeling well enough to see people. Once into the second and third day it had long been accepted that she would become very nauseous, sleep much of the time and be unable to cope with people. The first visitor to arrive was her form teacher, who talked about her friends and passed on the latest gossip from school. The deputy head, who had kindly kept in touch all along and had been very supportive and sensitive to our needs, also came a little later. We ended up talking about *Eastenders* and Jess famously joked about how she would never have thought she would have such a conversation with a teacher! Later that evening my cousin and his wife accompanied by their two young children, Sam and Ellie, arrived, and Jess was so very pleased to see them. She helped Ellie to draw a number of pictures and they really enjoyed each other's company.

It was refreshing for me too, as there was a lot to catch up on, and their visit rounded off a successful evening. Jerzy appeared later, tired from a busy day at work. I was very pleased to see him, as inwardly I knew things were not looking so good and I hadn't had a chance to talk to him since arriving at the hospital. After a short game Jess was so tired that she drifted off to sleep, so Jerzy and I took a walk up the corridor and I was able to take the opportunity to explain Nicky's findings.

Jerzy listened intently, absorbing our reality and sharing the disappointment I had quietly held within me since that morning. I guess I hoped he would reassure me Jess was going to be okay, but he couldn't, of course he couldn't. After the despair I had felt following the break-up of my first marriage, Jerzy had shown me a greater love, trust and understanding than I had ever imagined possible. I had been confident I knew what love was, but in retrospect I had no comprehension of it until I met Jerzy. He completed our circle; he completed me. He was the part of me that had always been missing and now he was there. He was an answer to my prayers, an 'angel' sent to help me and the children through, to ease our pain and support our needs during this most difficult of times. When Jess and I chatted quietly we often mused about angels, her belief was absolute: throughout the ages there have been references to angelic occurrences, situations and feelings that had no earthly explanation. Jess entirely believed that angels can gracefully, out of our awareness, intercept our experience and a person may be driven momentarily to do something that will change the lives of others hugely. I felt strongly, right from the beginning, that Jerzy and I were together for a reason. Our meeting had been quite random and yet our lives had changed beyond recognition. In Jess's world there was no doubt we had been introduced by angels.

Jerzy and I stood for some while in that cold, dark and uninviting corridor trying to process our thoughts together. We were still waiting to find out if radiotherapy would be an appropriate course of treatment for Jess and also I had contacted Mr de Ville de Goyet again to see if he had any suggestions for further treatment. I was unwilling to give up hope of a cure just yet. In light of the knowledge that Jess's initial response to treatment had been short lived, there seemed to be more of an urgency to pursue some further answers. Mr de Ville de Goyet had requested some up-to-date scan pictures so that he could make an accurate assessment and come to an appropriate decision, and we eagerly awaited news from him. For the moment we agreed to catch Nicky the next day for a further discussion on things and, as Jerzy had some work commitments in the morning, this would more than likely fall to me. Before he left that night he held me tight - he always said that by holding me close he was giving me strength to give to Jess. Whether this was actually how it worked, who knows, but it felt good for me to know that he was there, propping me up, and emotionally I couldn't have done it without him.

The next morning was the start of a very difficult day. Jess was in pain and feeling extremely ill. She was given the maximum doses of her anti-emetic medicine but she was feeling dreadful. She withdrew into herself, deeply depressed and clearly processing Nicky's findings from the previous day. Her depression was an established pattern but today she carried a new depth of despair, I wonder if she had suddenly recognised how she was possibly beginning to lose her battle for life. She knew that Nicky had felt the tumour more clearly the day before and I guess she was afraid. Coping with this extreme treatment was fine if you believed it was helping, but Jess had begun to doubt if it was doing her any good, and her will to continue started to subside. As she tried to sleep through her extreme nausea, I left her briefly to walk up the corridor. I sat on one of the chairs by the telephone and remembered my conversation with Jerzy in the same place only the night before. I must have looked tearful as many passers-by tried to talk to me, but I just wanted my own space for a moment. I suppose I wanted to cry but I hadn't wanted Jess to see me. I was concerned about so many things that it was hard to put my thoughts in order even though I knew I had to. In what seemed like only a moment, although in reality I could have been there quite a while, Nicky walked up the corridor. As soon as she saw me she knew that I would want to talk to her and in her usual caring and professional manner she immediately made time to accommodate that need.

Nicky led the way into her office and, as we had so many times before, we went over the facts surrounding Jess as they were at that time. She reiterated her findings of the day before and how she had always felt that the present chemotherapy was only ever going to be a holding measure. It was not the magic cure that I had still hungered for in my heart. There had also been some news from the radiotherapy department at Bristol Children's Hospital, which had confirmed that, although in principle radiotherapy was an option, the maximum strength of the treatment that could be offered would not be at a high enough level to cure Jess from this reoccurrence of her cancer; if the strength were increased to the required level, Jess would not survive the treatment. Thus it was strongly advised that this path was not appropriate.

Nicky had been contacted by Mr de Ville de Goyet who had come back with a suggestion of something known as radio frequency ablation (RFA), whereby a probe would be positioned inside each tumour and they would be burned from the inside. He had confirmed to Nicky that he would be able to remove the two largest tumours surgically and perform RFA on the two tumours buried deeper within her liver. This sounded positive until we looked a little closer at the facts. This procedure had not been performed on a child before, although the results of previous RFA treatment on adults had been encouraging. The problem was that, in order for the procedure to be curative, either radiotherapy or chemotherapy treatment would have to run alongside. It was not looking as though Jess would be able to tolerate further chemotherapy, not just mentally but also because her body was not tolerating these strong drugs. Her kidneys and her bone marrow were struggling. Nicky felt that further chemotherapy on top of what had already been agreed would not be appropriate for Jess, as the side effects alone were threatening her survival. In other words, she would more than likely die from the treatment rather than from the illness. We had already reached the decision that radiotherapy was equally as likely to end Jess's life, and therefore the initial excitement that Mr de Ville de Goyet may have come up with an answer slowly drained away, revealing the reality of Jess's dilemma.

Suddenly so much seemed to hang on Jess completing the treatment she was having, as there seemed to be no further sensible alternatives.

As Jess had been asking questions about radiotherapy and what was going to happen next, Nicky accompanied me back to see Jess, who was now awake and wanting to know where I was. I was totally unprepared for what came next - what parent could be? Perhaps Nicky knew from experience how this conversation would go and where it would lead, but this was completely new territory for me, so all I could do was listen.

Nicky started out by explaining the difficulties surrounding further chemotherapy or embarking on radiotherapy. We talked about the unlikely event of the present chemo having any lasting effect. We then talked about a possible operation in Birmingham, going through all the pain of surgery which Jess knew only too well. She was made aware that in order to bring about a cure she would have to have further chemo or radiotherapy, which she now knew was not appropriate. Nicky was so calm, talking to her in a soft, understanding voice but no longer reassuring her that treatment might bring about cure. This time she was giving Jess the facts. She had shown herself able to understand so much and Nicky had decided to tell Jess everything.

Jess listened to her every word, and tears welled in her eyes as she gradually came to understand where this conversation was leading.

"You're telling me I'm going to die, aren't you?" she said.

"Yes. I'm so sorry, Jess, but you are going to die from this tumour," came Nicky's response.

She went on to talk about the fact that Jess was never comfortable in hospital and that she could be supported and cared for at home if that was what she wanted. Moments of deafening silence punctuated the conversation. Jess was soaking it up and was now unable to say very much at all. It was so hard to comprehend all she had been through: the months of treatment she had endured; her huge operation; and her fight to return to school. She had been so very brave and now all that seemingly lay ahead was one path for her. Apart from the despair of hearing the words I had always dreaded, I remembered my initial promise to be there with Jess no matter what it took. I would never allow her to walk that last desperate path alone. Her bravery, trust and strength were exhausted and she needed the loving support of her family now more than ever.

After remaining silent for a while, crying and holding me tight, she suddenly said in a calm and decisive manner, "I want to go home. I don't want to have any more chemotherapy."The maturity of her understanding led Nicky to believe that she had to be taken seriously. She was saying that she wanted to stop her treatment fully in the knowledge of what that meant. Nicky questioned her on her understanding of what she was asking and the decision was taken to continue Jess on further fluid alone. The next lot of chemo was due to go up shortly and to delay that with some extra fluid would do no harm whilst we were left to talk. Nicky had to go and teach her students for an hour. I agreed that I would get Jerzy to come to the hospital during that time and we would discuss it all again when Nicky had finished her teaching.

Jess was firmly resolved in her decision. She hated hospital and had only tolerated it because she thought that the medical staff would be able to help. Now that she knew they couldn't, she didn't want to be there any longer than necessary. She was clearly angry and all I could do was to reassure her that I would always be with her and she would never need to feel alone. Perhaps I said the wrong things, who knows? It felt important to reaffirm our own strengths as a family and that Jess was very much a part of that and we loved her intensely. I didn't try to encourage her to continue; her decision had felt right. Even though none of us wanted to believe that she could die, this had been her decision and I respected that.

Jerzy appeared as quickly as he could and we went through the events of the morning with Nicky. He agreed that Jessie had made the decision and as long as it was all right with all concerned we would take her home. Nicky checked with another specialist who also confirmed that so long as Nicky felt Jess mature enough to understand her informed decision then we could be allowed to leave.

And so it was that Jess chose so bravely to finish her treatment.

Her lines were disconnected, she packed her things and she put herself in her wheelchair ready to depart as soon as possible. We said a final goodbye to those around at the time: the nursing staff who had kindly seen us through countless difficulties. Jess found it hard to do this and sped off up the corridor in her usual fashion. As she left the ward and let go of the wheels at the top of the sloped corridor, I remembered the numerous times she had done this before. Like a flight of freedom this had become her release and it had always been a truly happy experience. This time, however, she was sombre and tears ran down her cheeks. Anger and disappointment were written all over her face. In defiance, the speed that she reached on this occasion fuelled her mood and perhaps it was a release of the pent-up emotions she must have felt at the time. I was momentarily scared that she would do herself harm, but I let her go; she needed to do this and, sure enough, she slowed down with precision before the door to the car park. There had been no one around so no harm done.

Returning home, we talked about the Christmas play that was due to take place later that day. Originally Jess and I would have missed it, but now we would be able to attend. I knew Gemma and Stewart would be pleased and it was lovely that Jess would be able to enjoy something that would take her mind off the events of the day. Pleased to be home, she went to her room for a lie down, switching on her beside fan. Since receiving treatment for her illness she had developed a liking for air being blown at her face, and when she felt intensely sick it seemed to give her comfort. She put on some music and lay with her eyes closed, obviously thinking about the day we had had. I went to lie down also; I needed to cry and, unable to stop myself, I stayed in our room for ages. Jerzy stayed downstairs with Gemma and Stewart, who had seemingly not noticed that anything was different. I cried quietly, not wanting any of the children to know my sadness. I felt selfish for needing to do this - as though my feelings mattered! What about poor Jessie? She seemed to be coping so well and here was I completely consumed in my own fears. I needed to pull myself together, to be as strong as Jess needed me to be.

The light started to fade as this winter day began to draw to a close. The curtains were still open and I continued to lie in this half light, trying to stop my tears. The door opened with little warning and Jess came into the room. She wanted to know what was wrong - why was I crying? She knew full well what was wrong, but I suppose she wanted me to say how it was for me. I tried to diguise my tears but there was no pulling the wool over Jess's eyes that day. Through her trials she had matured beyond her years, possessing a gifted sense of intuition and genuine warm heartedness. It was clear she was feeling my emotional pain as I was hers. She needed to know and perhaps it was a good thing that she saw and understood how I felt.

"Mummy, I know you are crying about me. I don't want to die, but I just can't do this anymore. I can't face the chemotherapy and it wasn't doing me any good anyway, so there's no point in continuing."

Again she seemed so grown up, far older than her eleven years.

"I don't want to lose you Jess, I can't go on without you. I don't want you to die."

She hugged me, saying simply, "I know."

She was worried that I had been feeling cross with her for stopping the treatment. The reality was that she couldn't have been more wrong, as I had felt so very proud of the way she had coped and calmly come to this decision in her own way. We talked a little more, but I think we had reached a point where we both knew we could talk if we needed to but for the moment there was nothing more to be said. We needed to push on and ready ourselves for the school play as time was ticking by, so I pulled myself together and Jess disappeared to find something suitable to wear. I put plenty of make-up on to hide my puffy eyes and we set off to the village hall.

No one had been expecting to see Jess and I that evening, so it was hard to disguise the fact that the treatment had not gone as planned. I informed the headmaster that there was to be no further treatment, but I asked him to keep it quiet for the moment. We wanted to enjoy the evening as far as we could and, with Christmas looming on the horizon, I had to try to make sure that the children enjoyed things as far as they could. We had not told Gemma and Stewart about the events of the day and I had at least managed to conceal my intense sadness from them. It was not my intention for this to continue to be the case, but to have told them prior to the play would have been grossly unfair and I couldn't do that to them.

They were both extremely pleased we were all there. I sat with Jerzy, but Jess found a couple of her school friends and was clearly elevated by their company. We enjoyed the show as best we could, although inwardly it was hard to move my thoughts away from our dear Jess. Being with her friends successfully managed to distract her attention, but by the time we returned home she was visibly exhausted and feeling very sick. All the children went to bed at the same time. Jess normally wanted to stay up late but this time she was happy to find comfort in her familiar bed. Gemma and Stewart went to bed buzzing with the excitement of the play and the growing anticipation of Christmas. They were both pleased with themselves; they had each performed impeccably and done all that had been asked of them. I was very proud of them and it seemed unfair that they would need to know what was happening to Jess. I couldn't tell them at that point, but I would have to find the right moment. All my knowledge from reading information leaflets and books on childhood cancer had led me to believe that honesty was the only way to go, and children are far stronger than we give them credit for. The natural instinct to protect them from this upsetting news would be wrong and unfair in the long run. They both needed time to recognise that Jess only had a limited time left with us, and that she would die. I could not and would not deprive them of the right to find the strength to say goodbye in their own ways.

Jess did not sleep well. She was very sick and it was hard to get enough anti-emetic medication into her to control her symptoms. Due to her lack of sleep, she dosed off again whilst I was getting Gemma and Stewart ready for school the next morning. Jess had chatted with me during the night, the events of the previous day haunting her as she tried to sleep and the stress of this aggravating her nausea. Whether Gemma had heard our conversations or not I was never sure; maybe she had just picked up on various signals and expressions as we busied ourselves with the morning routine.

Suddenly she appeared at my side as I was preparing their respective packed lunches, saying, "Mummy, is Jess going to die?"

This directness can only be instigated by a child, a question placed with such innocent openness. I would never have wanted our news to be brought up so bluntly, but I wondered whether there would ever be a right moment and I couldn't lie. I answered her as openly and as simply as I could, saying, "Yes, sadly she is."

I then ushered her into the living room and explained as gently as I could how the treatment wasn't working anymore and that Jess had decided to come home from hospital. She was going to die but we didn't know when and we would take every single opportunity to make our remaining time together as positive as possible. I was going to make sure we had a lovely Christmas and both Gemma and Stewart would be able to help make Jess feel as loved and as special as we possibly could. Gemma cried, of course she did - I knew that the news about Jess would pull her world apart. However, I also felt strongly that to tell her, as I had, was the right thing to do. The moment had been dictated to me and she had understood completely all I had said. Stewart then appeared - he had been upstairs to find something in his room - and I repeated to him all that I had explained to Gemma, and in the same way that Gemma had done, he cried too. We talked about the things that we could all do for Jess, ways of helping her, and of course they both wanted to talk about Christmas.

Sooner than I would have imagined, Gemma and Stewart seemed content to continue to play although still visibly upset by the news. I couldn't send them to school that morning knowing how sad they were, so I telephoned the school to speak to the head again. I explained that I had broken the news to them both and I couldn't see how sending them to school would be a wise idea that day, feeling that we would be better spending some time together. He understood completely, being very supportive of my intuition, and prepared to follow my lead. He felt it would be useful to use this couple of days to explain the situation to the children at school so they could support Gemma and Stewart on their return.

Soon Jess appeared and she was wondering why her brother and sister were not at school. I explained that I had told them both about the day before and they wanted to spend some time with her. As she went into the living room I wondered what their reaction would be and how they would talk to Jess, or if they might choose not to speak about it. I decided to get Jess some breakfast and leave them to it. Only moments later Stewart came running into the kitchen looking for the Argos Catalogue and Gemma was anxiously searching for a piece of paper and a pen. Slightly puzzled by this I followed them back to Jess, carrying a drink for her. I don't know if I was really all that surprised by what I found, but Jess was positioned between them on the sofa and they were thumbing through the catalogue together. Jess was choosing Christmas presents that her brother and sister could buy for her and Gemma was anxiously making hasty notes on her piece of paper! They were laughing together and chuckled as they realised that I had discovered what they were doing. I knew instantly that my instinctive decision to tell them Jess's news had been completely right - we could all do this together.

Chapter 12

We now entered a new phase of completely uncharted waters. Jess's treatment plan had given structure, focus and, above all, a sense of safety. Now we were led by intuition, instinct and the fear of losing Jess. Although in the back of my mind for some while, this path was now our reality and would haunt me every waking moment of my day. What sleep I managed to snatch was my only solace, and in those midway moments between sleep and wakefulness, fear, loss and devastation would grip hold of me again.

Initially the relief of finishing her treatment, leaving the children's unit and returning home was enormous for Jess. She had found her most recent visit for chemotherapy hard to face and the thought of never having to go through all that again was fantastic. As the reality of her decision hit home, however, she became much more tearful: the realisation of her certain journey towards death encompassed her. Fear, anxiety and anger gradually started to invade the character of my beautiful daughter.

Death had initially seemed an easier option than continuing with the debilitating chemotherapy and she had faced this decision head on and with a maturity beyond her years. Behind the scenes, I was still looking into further surgery at this time, not entirely convinced that there were no more options, and Jess picked up on my investigations. I spoke to Mr de Ville de Goyet again, who had sounded keen to pursue the RFA path, although he did admit that without further chemotherapy or radiotherapy this would be no more than a palliative procedure. It would mean another huge operation, further pain and suffering for Jess, and being in hospital a long way from friends and family. Jess hated hospital, as she loathed being restricted and confined to one place. Knowing this made it easy to imagine just how traumatic the procedure would be for her. Then there was the question of whether she would indeed die during or shortly after surgery, as had been the biggest concern during her previous visit to Birmingham. He also admitted that if Jess were his child he would not know what to do, and I felt that, for a surgeon in his eminent position to say this, the hoped-for outcome of such a choice was by no means certain. Many of those involved in Jess's care clearly seemed to think that it was not in her best interests to go to Birmingham for surgery, although they were all very careful about how they talked about this with me. I suppose they felt it had to be Jess's decision and ultimately they didn't want to be seen to be influencing our thinking.

I came to understand how desperate Jess's situation had been right from the start and how it had been considered very unlikely indeed that Jess would ever survive. I couldn't recall anyone being completely that honest about her prognosis in the beginning, or maybe they had but I had only processed this information in terms of my own internal hopes. In other words, I could only believe in hope and to give up hope would have been to let Jess down. This was a time of re-evaluation, when honesty became more important than ever, not just in communication with the professionals but between Jerzy, myself and all the children. Instinct pointed me in the direction of complete honesty, a way of living from day to day that meant no whispering behind half-closed doors. Jess made decisions that were important to her, with Gemma and Stewart being encouraged to understand and know what was happening. We now knew of a handful of other cases worldwide - people with similar cancers - and no one had ever survived.

Right from the start of her treatment Jess had herself been aware of the unusual qualities of her illness and the chemotherapy was always done on a 'try it and see' basis. By the time we had reached this huge decision concerning the appropriateness of further surgery, Jess admitted that she felt like a 'guinea pig'. She felt that she was the means by which the professionals around her were learning and, although we were always hopeful that the treatment would work, Jess now felt that there was little in it to benefit her. However, she would often change her mind, switching from complete resolve not to pursue further treatment to wanting to venture to Birmingham for one last time, in a final desperate grab for life, which at best might only win her a few more months.

I think I always knew that this was it, but I just couldn't quite let go and I was always willing to sway with how Jess felt. Whilst she remained firm in her decision that was fine, but when she frequently changed her mind I felt I had to be there to support her. If ultimately she wanted to go to Birmingham I knew I would muster all my strength and go with her, supporting her in that decision. Likewise, if she decided, in an informed way, to stay at home and refuse further surgery I would support her in that too. What I could not resign myself to was denying her the opportunity if she felt that she wanted to continue and brave surgery one last time.

In writing about this decision it seems obvious that further surgery was not really a good idea and that Jess's quality of life was more important than trying to grasp at a few extra moments of time with her. But actually admitting that we had passed the final crossroads, that there were no other choices and that Jess had now begun her final decline towards death was truly the most horrendous situation any parent could ever have to face. I now realise that, in truth, there was no decision, only an acceptance of reality. I will never be able to express how difficult this time was. Complete helplessness engulfed my heart, but I knew that I wouldn't allow Jess ever to feel alone. I was committed to being with her and always walking alongside her.

Following Jess's decision to finish her chemotherapy, the team at the hospital continued to consider our care and support our needs wherever possible. This was difficult for them as there was no established children's community palliative care team at the time and so any help we received was very much about responding to the moment and employing the resources that were available to them. Following the initial diagnosis, we had had very little contact from our local doctors' surgery, despite the fact that a meeting took place between them and the hospital whilst we were visiting Hear'Say. True to their word, though, the hospital continued to help no end, with certain individuals doing all they could in sometimes quite desperate circumstances to support us. We were given a mobile phone number that we could call, day or night, and this phone was to be passed around the team in order to rotate responsibility for Jess's welfare.

Knowing that we could contact someone when needed was a big help. Jess's requirements had entered a completely new stage and I wanted to do all I could for her but had no previous knowledge to draw experience from. Her medication began to frighten me, as it became ever more complex and I was terrified of giving too much morphine when she was experiencing episodes of pain. Being able to ask for advice or call someone to attend was vital to my ability to cope but understandably became a huge drain on the hospital team and must have caused a great deal of pressure. I doubted my own abilities but knew that I had to be strong for Jess. She needed and had always trusted in my strength and I was determined not to let her down. I could not have supported her as I did without the commitment and strength of the team of people behind me, and I will always look back on this time with complete gratitude.

Christmas was approaching again and we decided to concentrate on making it as special as possible. Because the festivities of the previous year had been overshadowed by Jess's sad diagnosis, it became important to live for this moment and to give Jess something else to focus on. Looking back, I don't know how I continued from day to day, as my heart was breaking, but outwardly we approached the celebrations as every other family. We put up as many decorations as we could muster, particularly fairy lights, which Jess had always loved so much. Jess and I went on many shopping trips to buy further lights and other items to brighten up our sad home. She also wanted to make sure that she bought a special present for everyone she knew, which eventually she achieved. Even though she was extremely uncomfortable at times, her determination kept her going and she was so pleased with herself when she had completed this aim. On one trip Jess chose a fibre-optic angel, which diffused dancing beams of coloured light around the living room, radiating peaceful warmth to all. Jess seemed to respond to the therapautic qualities of colour and light, a reassuring warm sense of how she visualised heaven and I know this angel gave her a little peace when she sat in silence in the half light watching the changing colours. Every year Jess's angel continues this display at Christmas, reminding me of the peaceful, warm light that stretched out and touched my darling girl.

There was so much going on as the days before Christmas sped by that it was hard to make sense of everything and is even more difficult now to go back over that time with clarity. Jumping back and experiencing those thoughts and feelings and the emotional stress of caring not only for Jess but also the needs of our family, it is clearer to me now just what an intense time it was. Jess was greatly troubled by what to do, her thoughts swaying daily about possible surgery, and I tried to go with how she felt. I never wanted her to doubt my commitment to doing whatever it took to follow her wishes. This decision and all the questions and anxieties that accompanied her situation added to her stress, and her pain increased tremendously, often fuelled by anger, depression and fear. Night-times were by far the worst; she hated going to bed, sometimes completely overcome by the fear of not waking up in the morning. We continued to allow Jess to stay up late, which shortened the night for her and meant she would sleep on in the mornings. Initially she was reassured by hearing people about as they prepared for school and the day ahead, as it helped her to avoid so much night-time silence.

Evenings were spent playing board games or watching television. This was our special time with Jess, a very precious time when Jerzy was home as well, and we would try to experience some fun together. Gradually over these few weeks before Christmas, through the evenings her pain levels would increase until, by the time she was due to go to bed, she would be doubled over in pain, crying and terrified. Her fear of sleeping became worse, resulting in increasingly frequent panic attacks, and as a result she was prescribed tranquillisers to induce a calmer state.

Once in bed she would lie awake for hours, crying and lost in fear. Unable to leave her, I would sit on the floor by her bed and talk with her, sometimes into the small hours of the morning. We talked about all sorts of things, but mostly she wanted to talk about dying; she wanted to know what would happen to her. She was particularly terrified of choking, a thought that often haunted her. Unable to know for certain what would happen, I found it really hard to answer her questions, but once again honesty led the way for me and therefore I responded with my own views and beliefs in the hope that they might offer her some small amount of comfort.

Jess had chosen to accept Christ into her life and so she believed that in dying she would enter heaven and death was not the end. I believed that she would not only live on in spirit but also in the hearts and souls of those who loved her. In her anger initially she had turned away from her faith, feeling let down and lost. She believed that she had dedicated her life to Christ but that, as she had not recovered, he had not answered her prayers. As Christmas grew closer she still remained angry but less so with God. She rarely went to church (due to the discomfort of sitting for a long time) but she did believe, and during our late night conversations she often asked for forgiveness. This seemed a strange conversation to have but it was important to Jess. She wanted to go to heaven and she believed that she had been untruthful at times and told lies. She worried that if she did not tell me then she would not go to heaven. Several times we went back over this because I would say that there was nothing to forgive. I loved her completely and unconditionally. I explained how everyone makes mistakes, especially when growing and learning about the world. All these happenings are a part of our education, the learning process that makes us who we are. It didn't matter to me what terrible things she felt she had done; I would always love her and in my eyes there was never anything to forgive. These confessions were so important to her and, although I often felt saddened that such trivial incidents had grown into mountains for her, I listened to everything she wanted to say. I told her that without doubt she would be the brightest angel in heaven and she had earned her place in the kingdom of the Lord.

She often asked me what it was like to die and what heaven would be like. I could only answer with snippets of stories I had heard about people who have seemingly died and then been resuscitated. I told her how such people have reported seeing a light some way off that they have been drawn towards. I told her about an overwhelming impression of peace and being reunited with family members who have gone before. Unable to comfort her as a mother might normally comfort a child in pain, with reassurance of a brighter tomorrow, instinct led me to assure Jess that she had no need to fear death. I tried to describe how I thought heaven would be: a very special place, full of colour and warmth; a place of peace, love and understanding where she would feel no pain. She worried about meeting relatives who had died before her, as she thought that she wouldn't recognise anyone. I said that I felt she would just know who they were and everyone in heaven would be very kind to her. Inwardly I felt that the Lord had not deserted her at her time of need and that he would help her and would ease her pain, and ultimately she would be carried gently on her journey to an assured place in the heaven she believed in and visualised. Graciously I tried to walk this difficult path with my little girl, never wanting her to feel alone for a minute, but I knew eventually that I would have to turn back and finally encourage her to leave me.

I asked myself constantly whether I was saying the right things. I sought guidance from those around me but there seemed to be no one able to guide me or lift the weight of responsibility from my shoulders. How could there be anyone else who truly knew the weight of sadness I carried? But, even if there had been, I wouldn't have changed for one minute the special honesty that Jess and I shared.

We had some contact with The Rainbow Centre at Bristol who came to the house every fortnight to do some play therapy with Gemma and Stewart. Whilst they were engaged in play, I had the opportunity to talk with one of them. Previous contact with The Rainbow Centre had been very special and I hoped that these sessions would help both the children and myself to cope individually. I was so glad of the opportunity to talk things through and put things in order during this time, but we would often be interrupted by Jess before the time was up. She was encouraged to be a part of the play therapy but didn't want to join in, but also she hated the fact that I might be talking to someone else. She believed I should be able to talk to her about anything, just as I encouraged her to talk to me, and therefore I shouldn't need to talk to anyone else. It was true, we could talk about anything she needed to, but I couldn't weigh Jess down with how I felt. I was pleased to listen to her and help her find her way, but she found it difficult to accept that I, in turn, needed to talk to someone else. No amount of persuasion would encourage Jess to give me space to talk and therefore she would feel uneasy about these people visiting the house. Their appointments with us became another focus for her anxiety. She knew why they were coming and she understandably found acceptance of her situation very hard.

I really wished that Jess would find the strength to talk to this counsellor too. She had tried once and had actually found it beneficial, but after that she had declined any further contact. She was adamant that if she had anything to say she would say it to me and therefore I should do the same. I know she meant well; she wanted to support me as much as I wanted to be there for her. However, in reality there was no way that I could allow her to know how difficult it was for me, juggling looking after her, planning the best way forward for Gemma and Stewart, informing the schools, and keeping an open house for family and friends. There were also financial pressures, and Jerzy was carrying a huge weight of responsibility. He was working, but as he was self-employed he was unable to arrange much time off; otherwise we would not be able to afford to live and could end up losing our home. So much rested on his strength to keep going. He was my rock but he was feeling the strain. Visitors were the other element that added pressure and ultimately stress to my day. Knowing Jess's time was short and Christmas was approaching, many took the opportunity to come and see Jess at home. I therefore had to juggle visits from the hospital care team and the doctors, which were vital, with seemingly endless visits from well-meaning friends and relatives. In writing this, it sounds as though they were all unwelcome, which is most definitely not the case. I was pleased to see people; it was more a matter of lack of sleep and emotional exhaustion. I was up every night well into the small hours of the morning, and then I would be up early to get the children off to school. With our days packed with visits I would rarely have the opportunity even to grab a quick nap during the day. Housework didn't go away, and neither did the washing and ironing. I tried to limit some of my less important responsibilities in order to concentrate on Jess, but I rarely had the opportunity to relax completely.

My previous divorce meant that I also had to welcome members of Andrew's family into the house regularly. I recognised the importance of this time for Jess and I had always supported the contact the children had with their father's family, but it was hard for me inwardly to let go of past hostilities. I tried to be friendly and welcoming, but some of these visits were a huge trial for me. Sundays had continued to be the day when all the children spent time with their dad, and if Jess was well enough she would go too. Increasingly, however, she was unable to go out and spent much of her time on the sofa, and therefore visits from her father's family became more and more frequent.

Despite the imminence of Christmas, the house was full of sadness, fear, uncertainty and despair. I recognised the need to break free from this and try to raise everyone's spirits. If the weather was good and Jess was reasonably well I would keep Gemma and Stewart home from school and we would steal a day together: Christmas shopping, a trip out to the cinema or just staying quietly at home playing games, with no visitors. I remember one day I took them all to the local garden centre to see Father Christmas, a magical experience with live reindeer and other farmyard animals, such as cows, a donkey and some sheep. The queue was long but the children were amused by the surrounding animals, decorations, music and lights. Overall it was a totally enchanting scene, and although Jess had long outgrown tales of Father Christmas she was overjoyed to witness the excitement of her brother and sister. She played along with their childlike understanding and helped to add to their joyful anticipation of a forthcoming Christmas Day.

It was about this time that Jess decided that she no longer wanted to continue with her private tuition; she couldn't see the point anymore. I knew that these sessions allowed her to get involved with different projects and she was very intelligent and needed stimulation. But Jess felt she didn't need it anymore and it seemed like one more visit to fit in when we might be out having fun instead. I had valued her tutor's input into our day, she had been a great help to me, and I would come to miss her contact. Once again, however, I respected Jess's choice, and who could blame her? She wanted to make the most of her time and she didn't feel the need to learn anymore. I believed that she was the one who was teaching those around her with her strength of character and courage. I certainly learned a lot from her.

On 20 December Jess's condition started to deteriorate rapidly and her temperature rose dramatically, which was often the first sign of neutropenia. She had not completed the last course of chemotherapy and I had therefore not expected this to happen. A blood test revealed that she needed a blood transfusion and intravenous antibiotics. With Christmas only a few days away Jess refused to be treated in hospital and, in compliance with her wishes, the hospital team arranged for her transfusion to be carried out at home. There was concern that her condition could go downhill quickly, but they tried hard to enable Jess to remain at home for Christmas. We struggled for a couple of days to accommodate her wishes, but her health declined to such an extent that on 23 December an ambulance had to transport her back to the children's ward. She had an extremely high temperature, she had turned slightly yellow, she was shaking and her fingers and toenails were cyanosed. For the first time Jess had also started talking gibberish as she became delirious with her temperature. This was a dreadful sign and I was extremely scared for her. Never mind Christmas, this was incredibly serious and I felt as though everyone involved in her care was holding their breath - there was a real concern that she might not survive this episode.

Chapter 13

When Jess awoke on Christmas Eve in hospital she was bitterly disappointed. She knew that the doctors would make their rounds during the morning and come to a decision about how well she was. She had an air of determination about her that day. There was no way anyone was going to prevent her from enjoying Christmas at home. When I returned to her cubicle after taking a shower she said, "Mum, I know this is going to be my last Christmas and I want to go home. I have to go home." Of course I knew how important it was to her but the decision was out of my hands, although I do remember half joking with her about making a run for it quietly when no one was looking if I felt she was strong enough later that afternoon. She laughed at the thought of us scheming in this way, "That would be really naughty, Mum!" How we laughed. I could see her dimple again and that cheeky glint in her eye; I knew she had turned a corner. Actually I was perfectly serious, as at that point I would have risked anything to give my little girl what she most wanted for Christmas: the opportunity to wake up on Christmas morning surrounded by excitement and Christmas presents, with her family, and in our new home.

The intravenous antibiotics had clearly begun to work. I always carried a thermometer and therefore knew that her temperature had fallen drastically although it was not yet within normal range. She was still tinged with yellow and a little weak, but it was so like Jess to have turned such a remarkable corner; I had seen it happen before. If she really wanted something badly enough she would make it happen. The previous Christmas she had made sure that her chemotherapy finished in time for her to go home, and when poorly before her Hear'Say visit she had made sure that she was well enough to go. No one could refuse her determination and no one would have wanted to; she was a difficult child to say no to. She insisted on getting up, dressed and into her wheelchair, so that she was ready to go before the doctors came onto the ward. The nurses knew her so well and were not surprised when she asked them to make sure she was the first to be seen that morning. They knew that Jess had been seriously ill the day before and that her enthusiasm for leaving would not necessarily bear fruit this time, but they jollied her along.

Eventually her patience was rewarded and she was indeed the first to be seen. I remember how everyone laughed, as the first thing she said to them was, "I am going home today and you can't stop me!" Only Jess could have got away with that and it was a tough call to deny her. They examined her carefully and I remember a tense silence as Jess awaited their verdict. They confirmed how seriously ill she had been and pointed out that she was still in a vulnerable situation, but they also understood her need to go home. So, surprisingly, they negotiated a deal with her. She could go home for the morning and for lunch, but she would have to return for a scan at 2.30 p.m. followed by further intravenous antibiotics on the ward. If she were deemed well enough at that point, we could go home again. She would still need to return to hospital three times a day for the next few days in order to continue the course of antibiotics, but could remain at home between doses. This was a bittersweet victory for Jess. Obviously she would have preferred to leave and not go back, but she knew she needed the antibiotics. She also knew the doctors were being extremely lenient and this was a privilege she had never been allowed before. She therefore reluctantly agreed to their terms; after all, it meant she could wake up at home on Christmas Day.

The kindly nursing staff assured Jess they would have her intravenous drip set up and ready for her each time. The antibiotic treatment would only take 25 minutes to run through her line and they promised to hold her up as little as possible. The deal was only good as long as she remained well, but even if she had felt unwell I don't think she would have allowed anyone to know. And so, in her usual style, she was off down the corridor in her wheelchair and I had to run to catch her up in order to open the door at the end of the ward. With the door open, like a bird flying free from its cage she flew down the corridor again, propelled not only by the slope but also the excitement of Christmas. She had rebellion in her eyes and knew that she had got her own way to a certain degree. As I chased after her my eyes welled with happiness: we were going home; my Jess was feeling better and for the moment she had survived. Running her around for her medicine was no big deal if it meant she could be at home.

It would only be a few short weeks later that I would come to realise how lucky she had been to receive these antibiotics. Time was starting to run out and decisions about further appropriate care would be made. Because it was Christmas, Jess had been given a reprieve and astounded everyone with the speed of her recovery. After Christmas she was due to have a bone scan to determine her suitability for further surgery, and this would be her final chance to decide for definite. The antibiotics were a holding measure until the final decision had been taken, enabling us to have Christmas as a family and put off our indecision until the New Year. We had a chance to draw breath, to live for the moment and to delight in just being together.

That evening I again attended midnight mass in keeping with our Christmas tradition but this time, for the first time, Jess chose to come too. She was determined to go, to muster the strength to be there without her wheelchair and to brave the cold night air. I don't deny that I was concerned about this outing, especially in light of how poorly she had been and her continuing hospital treatment. However, life had gone beyond always remaining sensible and had become a quest for meaning in that moment. If Jess wanted to take communion on the eve of her last Christmas then I would do everything in my power to make that possible. This service was a poignant and powerful moment in our journey together. It was the first and the last opportunity for us to celebrate the birth of Christ in this way, as mother and daughter, joined by our faith and yet soon to be parted by fate. It was almost a sensory overload after our isolation in hospital: the candles, the decorations and crib scene; the carols sung by a full and enthusiastic congregation; the excited chatter of children in anticipation of Christmas morning; the anxious voices of family life making ready for the days of festivity; mothers with concerned hearts wanting to provide for the family to the best of their ability. All of my senses engaged in experiencing the moment not only for myself but also acutely attuned to that occasion being Jess's first, and also last. The local population were gathering, intent on finding prominent seats, a few of them aware of our plight but most of them blissfully unaware.

I thought about the worries and tension that I had experienced over the years, concerned about buying the right gifts and whether the turkey would be ready at the exact same time as the rest of the dinner. Now all that meant anything to me was just being with Jess, making her day special and simply rejoicing in our all being together. Jess wore the white fluffy coat and matching hat that she had purchased for her Hear'Say visit, and in the half light of this atmospheric occasion her slightly yellowy, pallid complexion was not visible to the outside world. She cuddled into me for support as we moved to find our seats. The lights of the Christmas tree reflected in her glistening eyes but she did not smile; her heart was heavy. On reflection I think she knew that this would be a last farewell. I held inwardly the sense of Christmas being about the joy of new life, but our reality was about accepting the moment and contemplation of parting. As I knelt next to her to receive communion I lingered a while to whisper a quiet prayer. Maybe God would hear me and already knew my aching heart. I prayed for her end to be peaceful and that she would feel no pain. I also prayed for the strength to continue to be constantly by her side in spite of my fear and gently travel this final journey with her.

As she received the sacrament I glanced sideways. Proudly she reached out to embrace the glistening silver chalice, closing her eyes briefly as she sipped. I remembered how she would often joke afterwards about the quality of the wine or not quite managing to get enough, but I sensed today would be different. She no longer seemed a child; she carried an emotional weight under which most adults would crumble, and still she smiled briefly up at our vicar as she gently withdrew the cup from Jess's grasp. As the magic of the Christmas choir rang in my ears she glanced back at me. For that instant in which our eyes met, I saw the joy resonating through her being and her proud sense of accomplishment: a moment snatched in time, but a picture that remains in my heart always. I was proud to present her before God that night and to be at one with her spiritual understanding. As hundreds heartily sang carols with the strength of their collective voices echoing around this majestic church, Jess's strength began to fail and her discomfort grew, along with my concern for her well being.

When finally at home Jess was proud of her achievement and visibly pleased to have managed to sit through the whole service. Her own strength and determination were still very evident but it had been a very long day; a day that had begun with the uncertainty of being able to return from hospital and had ended with what others may have seen as a 'foolhardy' mission to attend church in the cold night air with a desperately ill child. Jess was very soon in bed asleep, exhausted but also defiantly pleased with herself. She had won over the hearts and minds of the hospital staff and had completed her mission to attend midnight mass, and although she was in pain, to her it was worth it.

I want to write about the wonderful Christmas we had but actually it was tinged with sadness; of course it was. However, Jess fully appreciated waking in her own bed and enjoyed opening her stocking with her brother and sister. They laughed and joked and all three engaged in a joyous celebration together. Although very young, Gemma and Stewart knew something of our anxiety to get home for Christmas. It was almost a reflection of our desperation the previous year, and so they too rejoiced in our accomplishment. However, I was more prepared for Christmas this year. Jess and I had managed plenty of shopping - she never denied the power of retail therapy! Pushing Jess around the shops and engaging in festive activities had been therapeutic for both of us.

Today was the day that she would give her presents to everyone, special items that she had chosen thoughtfully and carefully, with a constant determination to keep shopping relentlessly until her task was complete. They were more than just gifts, they were a tender consideration for the future and also a part of her farewell to each of us. One gift that touched a heart string was that which she gave to Gemma. It was a silver necklace upon which was engraved the image of a guardian angel, and on the reverse side was a prayer that read:

Angel of God my guardian dear

To whom his love entrusts me here
Ever this day be at my side
To light and guard
To rule and guide, Amen

Jess was clear that she wanted Gemma to have something very special. She knew Gemma's high spirits and impulsive nature, which sometimes made her laugh but at other times irritated her intensely, and she was concerned about how Gemma would get on when she was no longer there to watch over her. Giving Gemma a guardian angel meant that she was always going to be looked after. When she found this necklace it was perfect. I remembered how Jess had been massively pleased with herself for finding it and Gemma was equally overjoyed to receive it.

The day was a flurry of visitors, presents and as much enjoyment as we could muster, interspersed with our promised visits to hospital. Jess resigned herself to keeping her part of the bargain, knowing that she was very lucky to have been granted this leave of absence in between her treatments. Our first trip to the hospital was filled with surprises. On arrival Jess found a present on her bed and her IV was all set up and ready to go, as promised. Sarah, a very welcome visitor, met us there to exchange presents. Jess loved her so much and it was wonderful to spend half an hour having a chat together. When in hospital Jess was generally placed in a separate cubicle with a glass window along one side. Isolation from the ward kept her safe from any infection, an ever-present consideration in view of her changeable immunity. Whilst we were chatting, suddenly an enormous Christmas pudding walked past this window, causing Jess to fall about laughing. This was closely followed by Father Christmas, and later on there were carol singers. The atmosphere on the ward was really special. Even Jess's IV stand was decorated with tinsel, and the staff clearly enjoyed making this Christmas Day a wonderful experience for all the children who sadly had to be there. Jess soon realised that it wasn't so bad having to return there. We were in and out in half an hour and, of course, she got to fly down the corridor three times in one day, so there was a positive pay-off!

Choosing Christmas presents was hard - what do you buy a

child who is dying? We decided to buy presents for her in just the same way as usual, although I knew the things she really wanted I couldn't give her: the gift of health, her future and happiness. She received from her dad a very special gift, one that I know meant a great deal to her. He gave her a star, which he named after her, and the package included a star chart and a certificate, which she proudly showed everyone. She would often look up to the night sky and ask where her star was, and in response I would choose the brightest star at the time and say, "Look, there it is Jess." It didn't matter which one it was; what mattered to her was that it was up there and it comforted her in a very special way.

A few months later I found a short piece that she had written about Christmas, dated 26 December 2001, which summed up the mood of the day from her perspective:

"Christmas was a complete shambles this year, although I got what I wanted. I had to go in and out of hospital 3 times that day just to have some poxy antibiotics even though I feel fine. Dad has bought me a really tear-jerking present - it's a star. I have a star of my own somewhere but I'll find it."

When I first read this I was overwhelmed with sadness that her experience of Christmas was described as 'a shambles'. I know I did all I could to make it as special as possible; however my resounding reflection of her illness as a whole will always be, "Could I have done more?" I also felt this was the point where her anger started to grow. I know she felt cheated of her future and jealous of others who would get to grow up and reach for their dreams. I was as close as anyone could be to her, and yet I couldn't possibly imagine how she managed to carry such emotional pain. I wished I could remove the emotional turmoil from her, but I couldn't. Her psychological pain began to grow in sync with her physical pain and the two would aggravate each other, fuelling anger and anxiety. They pushed and pulled at her psyche and gradually our happy, smiley Jess began to recede. Glimpses would shine through intermittently, but I think much of her energy was used in just coping with being. I was left powerless, along for the ride and completely helpless in her wake.

With Christmas over and her treatment done, we soldiered on towards the New Year. Again, all the anticipation of newness and fresh beginnings was a distant recollection of years gone by and certainly not what this was about for us.

Jess wanted to have a party. I was emotionally and physically exhausted and would have preferred a quiet night, but a decision was made to join Sarah and her family for an evening of food, fun and fireworks. Having not long lost her mum to cancer, Sarah would have preferred not to have had a party either, but she wanted to do her best for Jess and therefore happily agreed to host the event. I think Jess wanted to recapture the joy we had experienced together on New Year's Eve 1999, millennium night: the excitement of hundreds of fireworks, the noise and drama of the evening. This was 2001, only two years later, and who could have imagined the difference that such a short space of time could make?

Jess enjoyed getting ready with her make-up and glitter and there was a glimmer of the radiance that we knew so well. Her hair was attempting to grow back but she was less conscious of this now and, knowing that she was in trusted company, she was able to lower her guard. In other spaces she would remain self-conscious, hiding under hats wherever possible. Tonight she bubbled with the other children, brimming over with happiness to be there and amongst good friends. Sarah's four girls were an absolute joy, looking after her and including her in their games. Children have an amazing capacity just to go with the moment. Jess was there and having fun, therefore everything was great. I'm not sure if Jess was masking her fear as she danced and played or whether reality suddenly kicked home, but immediately after midnight and 'Auld Lang Syne' Jess became overrun with fear and through her tears she cried out, "I'm going to die this year, Mummy." A mixture of both angry and scared reared up and we had to leave quite suddenly in order to contain her emotionally. It was an abrupt end to the evening, but my instinct was to comfort her at home. It took her ages to go to sleep as her mind seemed to be working overtime, but her mouth was unable to transmit her thoughts. She was contained within her own walls of fear. I tried to reach her but realistically could only be alongside and offer comfort in the only way I knew how.

The next day was a strange one, almost numb and void of emotion. As individual members of a collective family we existed alongside one another, lost to some extent in our own thoughts but aware of each other at the same time. Tiredness had a huge part to play, and we lounged around and dozed on and off, comforted by the ambience of the Christmas lights. Jess's fibre-optic angel reached out and touched us all with her warm, changing splashes of colour. Jess kept herself very much to herself and often retreated to listen to music or watch television in her own room. I sensed that it was appropriate to give her some space, although I felt her pain and wanted so badly to lift this dark veil for her.

Eventually, as the winter daylight faded, I went to look for Jess. I knocked on her door and waited for her to invite me in, but there was only silence. I knocked again. This time I was acknowledged and gently entered. Her room was silent and in darkness. She was sat upright on her bed with her back resting against the wall. Through the failing light I could see a glistening reflection of her wet face, evidence of tears that had clearly flowed for many hours. She stared straight ahead, unable to alter her gaze, as I sat gently at her side. What could I say to her? 'Are you all right?' or 'What's the matter?' hardly seemed appropriate. I put my arm around her and hugged her tenderly, at a loss as to how else to reach her. Through this haze of sadness she said, "I was praying, Mummy. I was asking God to save me." She paused to choke back her emotion. "I want to live. I want to go to Birmingham for the operation. I don't want to die." We sat alone together in gentle silence for what seemed a long while. I held her close and confirmed my intention to do as she wanted.

Only the day before she had refused to entertain the idea of the operation and certainly didn't want the bone scan that would confirm if she would be suitable for surgery. Mr de Ville de Goyet had said that he would only do the operation if her bones were shown to be clear of cancer. Nicky had witnessed her wishes and felt that she was very clear this time in her understanding, and yet here she was, changing her mind again.

Standing back and looking at it now, it was a huge ethical dilemma and I feel sorry for those who were involved in it professionally. It wasn't easy for them but it wasn't easy for us either, and it was an understandably impossible decision for my darling Jess to make with ease.

The next few days were a continual mix of uncertainty that was finally resolved by Jess opting to stick to her original brave decision to decline the offer of further surgery and to concentrate on her quality of life. It seemed the only right decision, although extremely painful. Jess even took the brave decision to break her final choice to her dad. She wanted to be the one to tell him, effectively saying she was resolved in the fact she was going to die. He came to the house and they spent time alone together. I know she hugged and comforted him, she wanted him to know it was okay. It became clear that the uncertainty surrounding Jess's choice had prevented us from living, but now a sense of acceptance grew which enabled us to concentrate on making the most of just being a family, treasuring every moment of time we had left together.

The following is an extract from a letter from Nicky to Mr de Ville de Goyet:

"The family have agonised for several weeks about your offer of further surgery and radio frequency ablation. They were desperate for further curative therapy if possible, but Jessica made it very clear that she did not wish to have further surgery, and in fact decided not to have further chemotherapy halfway through a course in December. The Radiotherapy Department in Bristol had made it clear that curative doses of radiotherapy to her liver would be too toxic, and this was not an option they wanted to pursue.

In the absence of acceptable systemic treatment for Jessica, and the knowledge that further surgical treatment alone might result only in a local control of visible disease, Jessica and her mother have decided not to pursue any further surgical treatment. They remain extremely grateful to you for the operation that Jessica received in June, and have recognised that they had several months of good quality time in the summer which might not otherwise have occurred. The family are gradually coming to terms with the fact that Jessica's hepatoblastoma will not be curable and are focusing on maximising the quality of her

remaining time. They will be spending a week at our local Children's
Hospice next week.
Once again many thanks for your assistance, and for the hope and
support that you gave this family."

Chapter 14

As I busily packed our last few items and helped Jerzy load the car I was overwhelmed with the sense that this day had arrived too quickly. Were we really ready for this? Was Jess emotionally ready for this? I felt that we were taking a trip into the unknown and it was very uncomfortable, although outwardly I tried hard not to show my fear to the children. By contrast, there was huge excitement buzzing around between them; they chattered and bounced about as though we were off on a holiday adventure. In a way I hoped that this happiness would remain with them, as it served as a shield to their mother's unnoticed silence and protected them from the truth that lay beneath their joyous giggles. Jerzy gently comforted and offered a reassuring glance here and there as we worked together to get this voyage of new discovery on its way. He knew my pain, there was no doubt of that. He also knew that he could do nothing to help our situation other than to be firmly committed to supporting me to support Jess. By doing this he remained my rock, my connection to the ground, true and strong.

Eventually we set off. We were only going for four nights and yet the car seemed packed full of bags and excited children. Jess was outwardly reflecting the mood of her brother and sister and yet I wondered if inwardly she was nervous of what she would find and how it would be. She had asked many questions that I was unable to answer. I had a sense that we were going to experience the answers only if we were brave enough to make the journey. I wondered if the journey were not just the physical getting there but also an emotional journey of acceptance. It would take us about an hour to arrive at the children's hospice near Barnstaple in north Devon. The sun was out to greet us this morning and it would be a pretty drive across some beautifully stunning, rolling countryside, but my mind was elsewhere, lost in my own silence and deep within I reflected on the enormity of our emotional journey.

It was Monday 21 January 2002. The glorious day of our wedding had taken place on 29 April 2000. The weather had not been unlike today, crisp and fresh, and the warmth of our love had melted beneath the glowing spring sunshine into a sea of wonderful memories. The sunlight this day had the same quality but the splashes of light fell on a very different scene. How far away those precious memories felt from me today. Who would have guessed that we would have just six months together, united as a new family and blissfully unaware of our future, before being faced with the tragedy surrounding Jess's diagnosis and subsequent struggle to fight for her life. In June 2001 Jess had bravely faced surgery only to recover in the knowledge that she still might not survive. At this time I was quietly informed that she may only have another six months to live, but in disbelief we fought on defiantly together. And yet, here we were, almost six months to the day, making our first journey to Little Bridge House.

"Are we there yet," came a call from the rear of the car, a predictable call that every parent hears from impatient children anxious to be 'there' wherever 'there' was. We were not even halfway yet and when I conveyed this to them all three settled disappointedly back in their seats. I caught sight of Jess, who now appeared more thoughtful and was clearly processing this journey in her own mind. I asked if she was okay and was acknowledged with a simple warm smile although there were a million words contained in that gesture. I knew that I couldn't possibly begin to understand the enormity of the internal journey she was making. I sank back into my own world again and, as the countryside gently rolled past my window, scenes and experiences of the last few days flashed past in my mind.

Jess's decision to refrain from surgery had unexpectedly provided a sense of release for her. She no longer needed to gear herself up for more treatment, to watch the calendar, to dread the next blood test or indeed to do anything she didn't want to do anymore. But, having said that, we had no knowledge of how long she had left, we had no structured treatment plan from which to draw a sense of safety and her growing psychological angst had reached new heights over the last week. I was spending more and more time just being alongside her, with no answers to give or previous experience to draw on. My only guide was my honesty and I tried hard to encourage Jess to focus on that. She knew that up to this point we had shared an intense honesty and I vowed to continue that openness with her. In our long night-time conversations we explored the concept of hope. We knew that there was no hope of a cure, but we could hope for other things and I would never let go of the hopes we shared. There was the hope of shared happiness and experiences that we might still engage in; the sense that her journey was not yet done and we could find new hopes and dreams to focus on. My promise to Jess at the onset of her treatment was that I would never give up hope, but I guess we both knew that hope had changed its meaning. In acknowledging that we were still able to embrace hope, but perhaps in a different way, we could still hold the concept of that space between us almost as a light in the darkness of reality.

I suddenly awoke from my thoughts in a panic. Had I packed all her medication? There was so much of it now and I couldn't remember transferring this well-visited box to the car. Reassuringly Jerzy confirmed that he had done it and there was no need to worry. I glanced at my watch. I had become acutely aware of the time and Jess's next injections and tablets would be due in another hour. Of course I knew why I was so anxious about her meds - they frightened me. She was on some serious drugs now and in some cases large amounts, and by the time they were due she was ready for them. Delay meant pain and, if pain was allowed to grow, her anxiety would elevate and the pain then became difficult to control. It was a cycle that had fallen increasingly to me to monitor and manage. In some cases I consistently needed reassurance from medical staff at the hospital as to whether it was safe to give her more morphine when she was experiencing a peak of breakthrough pain. I was terrified of making a mistake. What if she died as a result of an overdose administered by me? At my worst moments of indecision and despair I worried about being blamed if I were to get it wrong. I also felt angry about this responsibility because surely I had enough to cope with, but I knew that if I always kept checking then I couldn't make a mistake. Sleep deprivation fed into my fear of 'getting it wrong'. In my tired state I could easily forget where I was up to with some of her meds. To keep it all clear in my head I drew up a spreadsheet of all her drugs, what they were for and when they were to be administered, which enabled me to keep myself safe. There is no doubt that my fear encouraged me to over-identify with this responsibility, knowing that a lapse in concentration could result in too much being given or not enough and she would experience pain. The idea of her being in pain was unacceptable to me, so I had to be acutely aware of getting it right. And so the cycle continued. Looking back, it was a behaviour that grew out of my wish to do the best for Jess and it was hardly surprising when you consider what was at stake if 'I got it wrong'. My mind stayed with the issue of her drugs as we began to draw near to our destination. Jess had been introduced to a drug that we knew as 'Actiq'. It was a product that could be sucked on and looked rather like a white lollypop. It was a powerful drug and I believe it came from the same group of medicines as morphine. There was no doubt in my mind that she experienced a 'high' from these sticks, but was that a bad thing when weighing up what she was going through? They were for her pain control but concerns had been expressed over why she was getting through so many. In her home-kept notes I had written the following entry:

"Hospital Pharmacy are questioning the amounts of Actiq Jess is having. I think that some is definitely for comfort, especially in the evening when she feels scared of dying and not waking in the morning. There have been a few days when I have not kept a note of everything mainly due to tiredness, although I have written down most of the medication given in order to keep some kind of record. Tomorrow I am going to count everything so that I can keep a clear stock list, as I feel that my integrity may be questioned at some point. I think this is unfair as I have been honest and open in every way about every aspect of Jess's illness. I have spoken to Jess about her answering questions when anyone asks her difficult things. Up to now I have helped her out when she has found it hard to answer, but I am not going to do this anymore as I don't think my answers are believed. I am trying to encourage her to talk more. As a family we have so much to cope with, it seems unfair that I now feel compelled to have to monitor Jess's medication in this way but it seems necessary. I will draw up some kind of form for keeping stock listed tomorrow, p.s. I am very sad tonight and I feel very alone."

146

We passed a sign indicating that Barnstaple was only five miles away and my stomach sank; I felt sick. What was this hospice going to be like? I had been clutching a booklet in my hand during the whole journey, trying to prepare myself. There was no doubt that I was afraid. We had seen so many sad things and witnessed so much despair, not just on the oncology wards at Bristol but also in Birmingham. It was enough for me as a parent to cope with my own distress without, as I had done before, trying to empathise with other parents. It might be like another hospital but this time it would be filled with dying children, insurmountable sadness and loss. These fears choked me and I had not wanted to go. It had taken much persuasion from Nicky, Jess's nurses and our wonderful social worker, to encourage me to agree just to having a look. My agreement had been that I would go on the understanding that if anyone was unhappy, and most importantly if Jess was uncomfortable, then I would pack and bring everyone straight home. Knowing that I had a way of escaping made it easier to contemplate. I looked at the booklet in my hand: the picture on the front showed a beautiful stone building and well-kept gardens, and it spoke of caring for the whole family and creating a friendly, informal and relaxed atmosphere. On the back it read:

"Little Bridge House aims to help and support families who face the emotional and physical strain of caring for children who, sadly, are not expected to live into adulthood. This does not have to make Little Bridge House a sad place, although sadnesses are faced together, Little Bridge House is a place of love, happiness and friendship.
We hope to provide a haven, a place where children and their families can be nurtured and cosseted, returning home with renewed vigour and a sense of anticipation for the next visit."

In my discomfort that paragraph reached out to me somehow: maybe these people would understand where we were at, but I would not know unless I gave them a chance, and the idea of "returning home with renewed vigour" sat well with me. And with that we rounded the corner into the driveway. As this magnificent building swung into view the January sunlight reflected off the stonework, giving it a warm yellowy glow.

There was little indication from the outside what lay within, only the initial sense that it was unlike any hospital building we had visited previously.

We parked in a courtyard by a central fountain, which was surrounded by bronze statues of children. They alone touched me: the curious expressions on their faces and the naturalness of their postures. I was reluctant to remove our luggage from the car; after all, we were not going to be staying anyway so there was no point. The children wasted no time in running to the front door, a beautiful stone-set entrance porch sheltering a large wooden door. I felt such a mix of emotions at this point, it seemed to take forever for someone to answer but, of course, in reality it was only the shortest time. In the waiting, however, I could easily have swung straight round and sought solace in the familiarity of our family car. Inside I was screaming and I'm not sure how well I was hiding that from the rest of the family. Jess seemed to have warmed already to this place and reflected the excitement of her siblings.

Soon the door opened and we were welcomed warmly and shown initially into the family living area, which appeared to be the heart of the house. It was indeed a warm heart and the experience of that alone moved me. This place was a home. There was colour everywhere and toys and families intermingled with bright, welcoming furniture and huge, cosy sofas - the type of seating that holds and comforts, made to melt into with a cup of hot soup on a winter's day. An enormous central stone fireplace dominated one wall and a piano sat in another corner. A home was not a home without a piano and here it was. There were meticulously intricate wall hangings everywhere, completed and gifted with love from dedicated friends of the hospice. Happiness, joy and laughter were evident on the faces of the children already at home in this house. My three were very quickly invited to join in and drawn off into a messy playroom where all kinds of activities were on offer. As they quickly relaxed with new friends so my defences melted, minute by minute. With each turn of a corridor or the introduction of another facility I felt my anxiety and fears recede.

The living area led out through a huge conservatory into a

magical garden with intermingled pathways and flower beds. Again, toys, bikes, trikes, diggers and tractors were spread around this fabulous outside space. Alongside lay a sandpit where younger children were delighting in the texture and possibilities of sand play. Dominating this scene was a little wooden bridge poignantly set amongst the twisting pathways. This bridge, for me, seemed to fit with our journey somehow. Perhaps symbolically it would be the end of the journey, the part that Jess would have to do alone. Maybe just the other side and hidden from our dimensional view was the heaven that Jess wanted to reach. Such was the magic of this garden that it would be easy to picture heaven existing just the other side of that bridge; voices of children laughing and calling, already departed from this world but offering gentle encouragement from the next.

We were introduced to Libby initially, who would be one of our own contacts, and who was a friendly and extremely warm character. She wore colourful well-fitted clothes and had mid-length dark hair, and she smiled a lot as she spoke to us, encouraging a sense of joy in our hearts. There were no uniforms or name tags and initially it was difficult to know who were staff and who were family members, but I soon realised that this added to the sense of family and informality. I'm sure we battered Libby a bit with questions, but she answered them all with grace, taking her time to be clear and dispel any misunderstandings or fears we were carrying. It was evident from the outset that this was a house full of honesty, which quite powerfully reflected my own instinct and ethos surrounding Jess.

Jess's medication was the first and perhaps the most significant responsibility I handed over. With trained nursing staff, a part of the care they provided was to lift this weight of responsibility from the shoulders of parents. There were regular visits from doctors for new prescriptions, with a dedication to watching the needs of the most vulnerable with extreme care. Pain management was a clear priority and if Jess needed some Actiq then she could have it, whether for comfort or not. The underlying principles were different here; it was about the care of the dying, palliative care. Jess was no longer receiving active treatment and therefore the emphasis had changed. Managing her pain would be a clear priority and knowing this meant that I could give myself permission to let go of so much anxiety - an anxiety that had clearly taken a lot of energy to hold. It was a moving experience for me and with it went my compulsion for being acutely aware of the time. I felt I could breathe again and enjoy the excitement of the children. The worry of 'getting it right' that had bound me in chains was removed in one gesture and I felt a sense of freedom to be me again. It was a huge inward shift that I know happened within a very short time of entering this special house and I'm sure it had a visible effect. Libby invited us to fetch our things and then she would show us to our rooms. Jerzy turned to me for confirmation that this was agreeable. Of course it was, although we chuckled together over my embarrassment for ever believing that it wouldn't be. I had been very wrong about this place and, although I knew very little about it at this point, I knew instinctively that Jess was going to be well cared for. As a family we were going to be held in a uniquely special way. We no longer had the safety of a structured treatment plan, but what we had instead was the safety of new-found family and friends offering warmth, friendship and love. Every minute soothed our wounded souls and it was pure joy to see enthusiasm and wonderment reflected in Jess's sparkling eyes.

The family accommodation was fabulous: en suite rooms with breathtaking country views across the fields and a beautiful mix of flower gardens and grassy spaces. Gemma and Stewart had a twin room situated quite close down the corridor, but Gemma was uncomfortable about the dark - a fear that had grown during Jess's illness. A lot of it came from the shock of hearing Jess calling out in distress during the night, voicing her fears about dying and terrified by her vicious hallucinations. I know Gemma absorbed some of this terror, but she managed it maturely and she was okay about sleeping somewhere new so long as she could have a light. Libby made it a quest to find something suitable and soon returned with a plug-in light that gently glowed in the shape of an animal face. Jessica's room was at the other end of the building with the other children's rooms, where the night staff could watch her and respond to her needs.

It was filled with interesting toys and a beautifully carved bed in the shape of a sea horse. The bedrooms were themed, so in 'Seahorse' there were lots of items reflecting the sea, such as cuddly sea horses, shells and books. On the wall above her bed someone had placed the letters of her name, which had been stitched in cloth and adhered to the wall. Seeing her name on the wall drew her into a sense of this being her room, her very own special space. She had her own television and the opportunity to do whatever she wanted without interference from her siblings. This was something that Jess joked about as being a good thing, but actually whenever they did wander down the corridor to see her she was always pleased to see them and find out what they had been up to.

The rooms had the potential to open straight out onto the garden and I could imagine the summer here being very special. With easy entry to the garden, every child could experience the joy of accessibility, opening up the potential for any dream to be possible. The care team gave me the impression that they were prepared to do anything necessary to make sure that we all had a good time and that nothing would ever be too much trouble.

The children quickly learned where everything was: the jacuzzi, the soft play, the games and toys. Messy play was a clear favourite with everyone and they enjoyed working with clay, painting and sticking. There was another room with a pool table, interactive games, musical instruments and even a drum kit. It seemed as though every single aspect of a child's thought process and play experience was represented in some way within these special walls. This first day seemed almost a kind of information overload. The children wanted to do everything all at once and would flit from one thing to the next, and so on, as though someone would take it all away before there was time to experience everything. Gradually we settled into a way of being here, which meant that we became a family again, with no worries about visitors, no phone calls, no work for Jerzy, and no housework or cooking for me and, of course, no medication worries and no eye on the clock. Gemma and Stewart particularly liked the idea of missing school for the week. We could just be together, having fun, experiencing new things and, most importantly, making some of our most precious memories. It was an oasis of calm, as though we had stepped into a new dimension where we were accepted and welcomed, and where there were no judgments or expectations, only each day as it came.

Mealtimes were signalled by one of the children being given the task of walking the length of the building ringing a bell. This was a job that Gemma and Stewart relished if they had the chance but it often caused an argument between them. I guess the care team had seen it all before and seemed adept at finding solutions (like another bell!) or negotiating for peace. The food was fabulous and as all the families gathered in the dining area at the centre of the house it was a chance to make new friends, to learn new possibilities and gradually to discover what a truly special place this was. By the end of our first day I felt that we were blessed to have found our way here. I was so pleased I had found the strength to step inside and trust in the possibilities that others had tried to explain to me but I somehow couldn't hear, or perhaps was not ready to hear. Now, here we were, together in the truest sense, among friends and welcomed in the warmest way. It was a soothing, reparative experience and this was only our first day!

Chapter 15

We were now in a room called 'Orchard'. Newly planted trees in neat rows were visible from the window, and I assumed they might be apple trees although I didn't know for sure. Between them were littered splashes of yellow and orange, early spring daffodils opening and reaching for the first rays of spring sunshine. They were very early - it was only 16 February, but there was no doubt they were there. As I lay on the bed holding Jess's hand I described what I could see. I knew her love of nature would have embraced this special sight. Long winter days filled with dark clouds and endless rain had prevented us from going out together countless times. Now that the sun was shining, there was a refreshing sense that spring was just around the corner, but dearest Jess was now too poorly to appreciate nature's miraculous changing scene. Still the seasons would continue to change, as they always had, but soon there would be no Jess. She lay limp and motionless, apart from her struggling, rasping breath. It had been three days since I had last seen the beautiful blue of her eyes; her lids lay heavy and she showed little awareness or ability to move. It was as though the pneumonia had banished her, quite suddenly, into a deep, almost unconscious sleep.

On this visit she had changed rooms a number of times, even having two rooms at once for a while. The care team was always pleased to meet her needs and come up with new suggestions in order to overcome her experienced difficulties. She liked Orchard; intended as an adult room, it had a double bed and en suite bathroom. It also held the biggest television, a clear advantage when you are eleven years old. She felt special in this room, perhaps slightly favoured in some way. She often joked about how she had worked her way into this room; she felt grown-up and privileged in this space. She liked the fact that I could sleep next to her and felt comforted by our closeness. For me, being always alongside had become all I could do now. We had been invited to return only ten days ago and Jess's decline had been dramatic during that short space of time.

153

I remembered how our first visit had touched us all, and how we had felt renewed and ready to continue our journey at home. Inwardly I had felt stronger. I had gained perspective, particularly in terms of Jess's medication, and had learned how to let go of this anxiety. Our focus and family outlook had changed. We had forgotten the emotion surrounding Jess's big decision and now concentrated on making the most of every day, although Jess's worsening symptoms meant that it was not always possible to leave the house.

One day I had managed to take Jess and a friend into Taunton shopping. I stayed close and manoeuvred Jess's chair, and intermittently she would walk around with her friend, Kylie. They enjoyed trying on clothes together, laughing and joking, and it had been really special to watch them enjoying this girlie time. I had a real sense that Jess was starting to accept her changed appearance and was becoming less self-conscious in front of her friends. Spending time with Kylie in this way was a real celebration of who she was; she revisited her love of fashion and delighted in sharing this with her best friend.

After lunch in a fast-food restaurant we dropped Kylie off and I took Jess to the hospital as requested by Nicky. Whilst waiting for her to meet with us Jess had fallen asleep on the hospital bed, exhausted from her trip. She was in pain but felt it was a fair trade for the fun she'd had. Nicky spoke gently to me as Jess slept. There was little doubt in her mind that Jess's symptoms were worsening. The tumours, which initially had been difficult to locate, were now very palpable and her bloods had begun to change. Gradually the bilirubin levels had begun to climb, although there were no visible signs of jaundice at that time. I don't think it was that much of a surprise. I knew things were becoming more difficult and she had taken to sleeping for much longer spells. There was never any indication of time, however, and I was glad not to know as it was easier to tell Jess I honestly had no idea. We had spoken for a while about a possible trip to Paris and this had been organised. It was only a few weeks away. Jess's grandparents had paid for her, Jerzy and myself to travel by Euro Star and stay in a hotel near to the Arc de Triomphe. Jess was very excited about this trip and often teased Jerzy about the Eiffel Tower and his fear of heights. Now, however, it was becoming increasingly difficult to see how we were going to be able to do this trip. We were starting to look at the possibility of taking a member of the nursing team with us. I had been unable to organise insurance and there was a real worry that her condition might become critical during the trip and we would be stuck a long way from home. Jess's enthusiasm and hope for this new experience had encouraged me to try as hard as possible to make it happen. But gradually this particular hope was becoming an impossibility, which was finally sealed by dramatic changes in the management of her symptoms.

Part of Nicky's discussion surrounded the issue of changing Jess's medication, which had mostly been in tablet form with limited use of her central line. Jess had been experiencing stomach pains, sickness and a general intolerance to some things. The plan, therefore, was to move her across to a syringe driver, which would release measured amounts of meds directly through her line, bypassing her troubled stomach and travelling straight into her bloodstream. Being on a syringe driver would be a permanent arrangement and would certainly mean that Paris would no longer be possible. I dreaded having to break this news to Jess. It would mean her returning to the hospice so that this transition could take place in a medically controlled environment. No timescale had been set for this and there was a sense that, by continuing to manage as we were, we might be able to delay this next step for as a long as possible. As we drove home from the hospital Jess felt every bump in the road and with every turn of the car her discomfort was apparent to me. If travelling this short distance home was so uncomfortable, how could we realistically contemplate a trip to Paris?

Hours drifted by as I stayed by her side. Sometimes I dozed myself. Sleep had become difficult in long stretches, as my own body clock had become much attuned to Jess's needs. I would remain acutely aware of her breathing, which became erratic from time to time. I would hold my own breath in fear, waiting for her to resume her steady, rasping rhythm once more. Sometimes a member of the care team would arrive and listen to Jess's heart, take her temperature and monitor her breathing. Afterwards they would offer me the opportunity to talk, always empathic and full of compassion. Sometimes words were not appropriate and were replaced by silent, gentle hugs and the opportunity to share a tear.

Every so often I would attempt to introduce moisture to Jess's mouth with special sponges. I couldn't remember the last time she had drunk a glass of water. I talked to her about whatever came into my head, but often I simply lay there in silence, cuddled up to her and holding her hand. I hoped that she would know I was there, as I had promised I always would be. As I lay at her side, watching her every breath, my gaze wandered over to her syringe driver, standing purposefully on a stand by her side. It did quietly administer the drugs that kept her comfortable, there was no doubt about that. It silently pushed a syringe that held a concoction of morphine, anti-emetic drugs and something else to help her feel calm. Managing her symptoms at home had rapidly become traumatic and this instigated our return to Little Bridge House, in order to get things under control again. I knew that this would mean the introduction of the syringe driver and with it the final recognition that Paris was no longer an option. Jess had been devastated, as focusing on this trip had kept her going, given her something to aim for. She had lost the joy of hope and now there was nothing, from her perspective, but being attached to a machine all day. The care team had been marvellous, looking for other excitement to add that extra something into her world. In her sadness she even declined a visit from Noel Edmond's, organised in the hope of filling some of the void that Paris had left in her heart. There was no doubt about it, Jess was struggling to come to terms with this profound change. She was not a stranger to a syringe driver, but in the past they had been temporary whereas this was permanent. They had even served to measure time until her chemotherapy finished; half a syringe or less meant that we were nearly done. Now when a syringe finished another would be set in its place; a continual cycle, and one that she would never experience ending.

For a few days Jess could still wander about, trying to join in here and there, although increasingly her energy was ebbing away and her appetite had begun to dwindle. The food at Little Bridge House was wonderful and the staff would make Jess whatever she wanted, even if she could only manage a few mouthfuls. She never lost her love of chocolate, however, and was particularly fond of the chocolate mousse, which she rarely needed encouragement to finish. Her brother and sister ran around the house engaging in whatever they could find to do and supported by a watchful care team. Their enthusiastic energy never seemed to diminish and as I was spending every moment I could with Jess I was unfortunately no longer aware of where they were or what they were doing. Orchard was at the end of a long, winding corridor and every so often I would hear little feet running towards us, getting louder and louder until they arrived excitedly in our room. There would be a sweaty Stewart, who had spent ages messing around in the soft play area and letting off steam with other children and was anxious to tell me all about it. Intermittently Gemma would appear with yet another plateful of chocolate brownies which she had baked, or her speciality - chocolate pie! With each change of shift came new enthusiasm for doing the same task over and over again, which Gemma experienced as delightful. Other families were always keen to sample her efforts and she was happy to please. So these intermittent visits from my younger children brought bright spontaneity and news of the house to the declining truth in Jess's room.

Gradually, over the course of this visit, Jess had begun to spend more and more time in her room and rarely left her bed. Staying with her meant that gradually we both became more isolated from the rest of the house. I would hear the bell being rung along the corridor at mealtimes, and if Jess was asleep I would venture up to the living area to join with everybody else for something to eat. It was refreshing to experience the normality of family existence just for a moment, as though stepping aside from reality into a parallel dimension. Here our situation was accepted and supported. Every parent recognised our agony as a journey each would have to face in time, but in our shared awareness they offered a sense of new-found family strength.

I remembered how Jess and I had still managed to go in the jacuzzi every evening after Gemma and Stewart had gone to bed. This was a special time that we shared, with music and coloured lights floating randomly around. Jess particularly enjoyed the support of the water, soothing and relaxing, although her time here would be limited by her pain levels. In order to go in the water she would be disconnected from her syringe driver, and as soon as the pain became too great we would have to leave. It became a rush to get her back to her room and onto her pump again, and then almost immediately she would drift into an exhausted but medically soothed sleep. She looked forward to the jacuzzi, her love of water with her to the very end, but gradually this too became hard to manage. I will always remember the last time we were together in this way. Jess had asked our carer to put a CD in the player which she had bought me for Christmas. Tonight was different. She was no longer able to tolerate the bubbles but instead floated motionless on the surface of the water. I supported her head on my shoulder and together we listened in silence to the gentle voice of Eva Cassidy. There were no words for this time; it was a moment when silence said it all: the stillness of the water, the drifting coloured lights and the warmth of the love that bound us both in her journey. I believe that Jess knew this would be our last time, her final grasp at being with me again. As the music came to an end she said simply "I love you mummy, you've done so much for me". She waited until the end of the music, perhaps a little too long in hindsight, and by then it was clear that she was in intense pain. I struggled to lift her from the water and get her back onto her pump. Her decline was dramatic and just in that last 24 hours there seemed to have been a huge change.

As she lay with me now, noisily peaceful, it seemed unbelievable that she had managed a visit from Sarah and the girls just a few days earlier. Jess's excitement had been unsurpassed, and the girls were a delight and were made very welcome by everyone in the house. They played in the soft play, enjoyed the jacuzzi and even played pool together. Jess moved around tentatively, reluctantly pulling her pump along and unable to bend down in order to lean over the pool table, but she found ways of keeping up and managed well, her old determination shining through and genuinely extremely pleased to see everyone. I remembered her beautiful smile and, although her eyes were less bright, they nevertheless reflected the joy expressed in her heart. I loved their company too. Sarah was a treasured friend, and I really valued this visit and will never forget it. After this day we would never be together in the same way again and Jess would leave a void in our ability to be together which would never heal. I now know that losing Jess and my subsequent grief changed me profoundly. Relentless emotion would wash over me with seeming unpredictability and nothing would ever be the same again. Somewhere in the turmoil of this cycle of loss Sarah and I grew apart and, devastatingly, I eventually came to lose my dearest friend.

Our stay this time had been longer than intended and it was now clear that Jess was not well enough to make the journey home. Little Bridge had become our haven where we could just be together and recharge our batteries in readiness to receive friends and family when we were home again. But things had changed quite drastically over only a couple of days and sadly Jess had developed pneumonia. Her dad visited just before this diagnosis became apparent and he sat on her bed chatting with her for some while. I remember her sitting up to give him a huge hug as he was leaving, and he gave her a beautiful bunch of roses which remained by her side as she drifted into a deep sleep very shortly after he had left.

The next day she had woken up with a sudden energy, determined to send a present and card to her boyfriend for Valentine's Day. Where this sudden spurt of ability came from I shall never know - perhaps it was sheer determination to complete that which needed to be done. She miraculously got up and dressed and insisted on being taken to the village shop where she bought him a special gift and chose two cards, one for Craig and a birthday card for his sister Kylie. She insisted on walking round the store even though she was weak and unsteady on her feet, so I followed her around, afraid that she would fall but trying to support her very strong impulse to complete this incredible mission for both Craig and Kylie. On our return, she wrote both her cards and instructed me to post Craig's present and card in time for Valentine's Day. Kylie's card, once completed, was placed by the side of her bed with an instruction to post it in time for her birthday. Then, with her mission complete, she drifted again into a deep, unwakeable sleep. That was the last time she had spoken or opened her eyes. The next day a bouquet of flowers arrived from Craig. I described them to her, placing them in a vase next to her bed, and I'm sure she knew they were there. This was a relationship that had developed in primary school and I wondered about the future that they might have had together. Jess's determination to mark Valentine's Day was a measure of the depth of affection she felt towards him and a potential future that was a deep loss to them both. The flowers were a touching gift from a very dear and constant friend.

And so she had remained deeply asleep these past few days. I had played her music, read her poetry and also begun to read from *The Lion, the Witch and the Wardrobe* by C.S. Lewis. I was encouraged to believe that she could still hear me and so I continued to talk to her as though she were fully awake. Describing the multitude of daffodils and all I could see from the window was an extension of the need to keep her engaged, to be heard, and for her not to feel alone. Wherever her mind was, if I kept talking and stroking her hand she would know she was not on her own. As I read about Aslam, with his beautiful glowing mane, walking quietly towards the stone table I wondered if Jess was there too - knowing that she was going to die but accepting that her journey was now almost done. I felt like one of the girls, perhaps Lucy, walking gently alongside, not knowing what was happening and powerless to make a difference. Orchard was situated next to the chapel at the end of the building, and outside the chapel was a newly completed garden based on *The Lion, the Witch and the Wardrobe*, and this had been my inspiration for beginning to read this story to Jess. Not many days earlier she had played in this garden, with its twisting colourful pathways, sounds triggered by sensors, musical chimes and fountains. Jess loved it, and entering through the huge wardrobe door had been a complete delight to her. Perhaps she remembered this garden as she listened to the words of the story. It was not unusual for me to read to her, as often when she was too ill to concentrate on the words for herself I had read to her in hospital. It helped to take her mind off her sickness and projected her to another place, far away, where children could be children and there was no illness or pain. I continued reading in the hope that I was lifting her away from this room and engulfing her in childhood fantasy once more.

Throughout her illness, her treatment and her relapse Jess had been responsible for making many decisions. We had talked things through but ultimately she made the choices - informed choices that she perceived as being in her own best interests. Pneumonia had developed quickly and had left her unable to speak, so suddenly Jess was no longer able to make decisions and I was left trying to do what I saw as 'the right thing'. The situation that weighed heaviest on my mind was the fact that everyone back home was expecting us to return home the next day, Sunday. I had made the decision not to tell people that Jess had become so poorly. For a few hours there had been a glimmer of hope when there was a slight improvement in her breathing. Maybe she had tried to fight it for as long as she could, but now there was no possibility that she was going to survive this episode. We were certainly not going to be able to go home. Jess loved this place and it was as though she had chosen to stay. If her family knew she was so close to dying I felt that they would want to be there, but a part of me wondered who that would be for. I remembered how, when watching a film in which a character was dying in bed surrounded by a roomful of people, Jess had said to me that she didn't want everyone stood around watching her and waiting on her last breath. The last visitor she had had was her daddy, who would remember their last goodbye and giving her the roses that still adorned her bedside. And so I decided to keep our gentle space together. Although I felt very guilty, I also knew that I needed this time just to be alone with Jess. Jerzy and I discussed this decision and the care team agreed. I just hoped that people would forgive me.

Sunday continued in much the same way as the days before. I stayed with Jess constantly, often wondering how long she could go on like this. She lay slightly elevated with pillows with her head listing to one side and no amount of trying to change her position seemed to help: her head always sank to one side with her chin resting on her struggling chest; unable to move or make contact with the world around her and lost somewhere in a deep sleep. She had a high temperature, which gave her a pinky complexion in contrast to the gaunt yellow of previous times. As I continued to read to her there were more moments when she would stop breathing and I would find myself willing her to stay just a little bit longer. I wasn't ready for this; there was something in me still hanging on - perhaps it was our old friend hope still holding an active space between us.

Jerzy had taken Gemma and Stewart out to a local theme park and eventually they arrived back excitedly bearing gifts for Jess. The night before I had gently explained to both of them that Jess had very little time left and encouraged them to know that it was time to say goodbye to their sister. Although they had enjoyed their day out, they had both clearly thought of her and wanted to buy her a gift each. Such was the atmosphere at Little Bridge: they were able to enjoy the excitement of the house, a day out, or a special activity and then wander down the corridor and know intense sadness. Over these few days they had wandered in and out of her room; like little rays of sunshine they would appear and then be away up the corridor again to play. It was like jumping in and out of puddles: from sadness to happiness and back again. They jumped in and out of our journey, catching enough snippets to know the truth of their sister's deterioration.

As Gemma and Stewart went to bed they both gave their sister a kiss and a hug, each knowing and remembering my words from the previous evening. I said goodnight to them too. I didn't want to leave Jess that night and Jerzy was happy to put the little ones to bed. Soon he returned and we sat quietly by Jess's bed together. Every breath she took seemed to be a struggle and noises bubbled from her chest with rasping effort. It was heartbreaking to see her this way, lost in a deep sense of unconsciousness, and I could only hope that she could feel no pain. I sat up with her until about midnight, when my eyes could no longer stay open, and then laying next to her I fell asleep, although continually aware of her breathing.

Suddenly I was conscious of someone in the room. Opening my eyes I focused on Maria, one of our nurses, who had come to check Jess's pulse. She gently informed me that Jess's condition had worsened: her pulse was very fast and poor Jess looked as though she was really struggling. I cuddled up to her and held her hand, knowing she couldn't possibly continue in this way for much longer. Eventually her breathing suddenly changed and Maria disappeared to go and find Jerzy. Whilst we were alone something changed in me also. I couldn't bear to see her this way and I think we both let go of our hope at the same time. I told her that it was time for her to go and be with Jesus now, and that I would always love and remember her. I held her in my arms and sang to her quietly through my tears, as I had when she was a baby:

Be near me Lord Jesus, I ask thee to stay
Close by me forever and love me I pray
Bless all the dear children in thy tender care
And fit us for heaven to live with thee there

What seemed like only moments later Jerzy and Maria returned and Jess took her final, long drawn-out breaths. As she passed peacefully away, Maria kept checking her pulse and when she could hardly feel it anymore she quietly whispered, "Go gently, Jess."

Chapter 16

And so a gentle silence fell over this room. No longer was Jess struggling for breath, as in those moments she had left this world. I wondered if her soul had been led outside to that little bridge that stood so prominently in the garden and had welcomed my curiosity when we first arrived. Maybe she had been greeted as she walked tentatively across, warmly welcomed into heaven by other children who knew her journey: the heaven we had often talked about where children could be children, full of colour, warmth and love; where she would know peace and there would be no pain.

I continued to hold her for some while, drowning in sorrow and reluctant to move from her side. Maria and the other night staff were marvellous. There was no hurry. They compassionately supported us in our loss and encouraged us to take all the time we needed. I made only one phone call myself - to my special friend Sarah. It was only just after four in the morning, but I felt she would want to know. Jerzy continued with phoning family while I remained with Jess. Maria encouraged me to help wash her down and to change her clothes one last time. She remained warm to touch although lifeless in her expression and her chest no longer struggled for breath. As I disconnected her syringe driver from her line I felt as though at last she was free - not just free from the physical pain and her diminishing abilities, but also from the psychological pain that had bound her; the pain of knowing she was dying. She was no longer trapped inside a failing body on this bed where she had laid for days. She was my angel now and I hoped with all my heart that she had found the peace she deserved.

Whilst I continued to attend to Jess with Maria's help, Jerzy went outside and stood by the garden looking up at the stars. He had come to love Jess as his own, he knew she loved him too and he felt her loss as I did. By the time he came back inside, Jess was now at rest with all medical evidence of her struggle removed from sight. We sat at her side weeping together and drinking tea as morning began to approach. Jess needed to be moved at some point to a special room called 'Starborn', situated just across the corridor. Starborn was a beautifully peaceful room, reserved for those children who had died. It was just like any of the other bedrooms except that the bed housed a special cooling device. I remember my heart sinking as we sat quietly at Jess's side and I heard the cooler being switched on. It was only a gentle whirring, but in the silence of these early hours it could be heard clearly; subtle but necessary preparation to care for Jess's lifeless body.

I felt that it would be best to leave the nurses to move her whilst Jerzy and I went to break the news to Gemma and Stewart. They woke the instant the door to the room opened. I think they knew by my face before I spoke the words and we all cried together. The family room we now occupied had two single beds and a double bed in the middle. We all four sat on the double bed and between us all we remembered happy times together, special moments that stuck out or came to mind at that moment. I encouraged them both to know that they could hold their memories and that we would never forget their sister. They talked about the ways they would like to remember her and Stewart was very clear about lighting candles. He had always said, even to Jessica, that he wanted to remember her by lighting a candle at special times. And so we began a different journey, one that held Jess's memory at the centre, but we had to continue as best we could on our own.

By the time I had showered and we went back downstairs it was light outside. I went straight to see Jess, who was now laid out in Starborn. As I opened the door for the first time, the coldness of the air struck me instantly, but in spite of the physical cold the room held a gentle, honest warmth - the same honesty that led me always to speak the truth to the children, and the same honesty that echoed through the walls of this special place; nothing was a secret, everything was shared. I knew that Gemma and Stewart would not be shielded from seeing their sister in death and they would be gently supported and encouraged to see her when they felt ready. I remembered how, on our first night in the hospice, a little boy had died suddenly in the night. Through that first week I had witnessed from a distance his family being supported and his younger brother and sister freely wandering in and out of Starborn, speaking to him and loving him as though he were still alive. Their mother would accompany them both to say goodnight to him at the end of the day and they could spend whatever time they wanted just being with him, quietly accepting his passing. Speaking with their mother later in the week had been an inspiration to me, and I don't know if she ever knew just how much strength she gave me. Her shared honesty alone enabled me to know that I could travel this same path guided by the compassion and genuine holding of the care team. I knew that Gemma and Stewart would be well cared for, understood and guided through this most devastating of times. I wondered if Jess was caring for us by choosing to die here. She must have known that we would be well held, almost cocooned and protected from the outside world, held in the grace of our own experience.

Jess was laid out on this little carved wooden bed. She looked quite different now. Her skin had cooled and she no longer reflected the flushed appearance of her fever. She looked beautiful, like a china doll, her complexion perfectly smooth and clear. There was a slight smile on her face and a sense of her finally being at peace. I sat by her side once more and held her hand again. It no longer wrapped loosely and warmly around mine. Her whitened fingers seemed brittle and cold, fragile and strange to the touch. She no longer felt like my little girl; her body was now a cold shell, a shadow of the memory she had left behind. Very soon Gemma came in to see Jess. She was fine, a little nervous initially but keen to help me decorate the room. Stewart chose not to see Jess and tried hard to stay away, preferring to continue with the play he had known over those last painful days.

We decided to surround Jess with fairy lights. She had been disappointed when the Christmas decorations had to come down at home. The staff at Little Bridge set about finding some lights for us just as various family members started to arrive to see Jess, so it became a joint task to put them up. I was sat next to Jess talking to Andrew when Stewart stuck his head around the door looking for his dad. He was quite shocked when he caught sight of Jess and quickly disappeared again. It had happened by accident that he saw her and he definitely remained away after that. He never seemed to be unduly upset by this experience and a few years later he said that he was pleased he had seen her but that was enough for him. Gemma seemed happier to come in and out, bringing a growing collection of cuddly toys and placing them at the end of her bed. Andrew's roses were placed by her, now wilting slightly but helped by the cooled air. Gradually other flowers arrived, helping to decorate and fragrance the room.

This first day as I greeted people I found myself reliving her death over and over again. Still carrying the guilt of our decision not to warn people of her decline, I wrestled with explaining myself. Perhaps I didn't need to; maybe it was my own anxiety that led me to feel that an explanation was necessary. I felt I owed people an apology, although not one person gave me a hard time about it. I suppose deep down I wanted confirmation that I had done the right thing, that I had made the right decisions when Jess was no longer able to guide me. I felt lost in a void without her, struggling to swim in her wake but completely adrift in a sea of grief. Outwardly I have no doubt I gave the impression of coping well, but inwardly I was completely lost. I remember often having the sensation of struggling to breathe, almost consciously having to think about every breath I was taking.

I know that Jerzy became worried about me and later in the day, advised by Jess's doctor, he took me for a walk around the garden. We sat together quietly in *The Lion, the Witch and the Wardrobe* garden. Today was the day we would have been returning together from Paris, the trip that Jess had so looked forward to. We reflected on this and how quickly she had declined once it was certain that she could no longer go. It seemed poignant that she had chosen today to make her own final journey, I felt sure that heaven was a better place than Paris anyway. Jerzy knew that I had been repeating myself over and over again and he wanted to break this cycle and remove me from the situation. He was so right to do so. He reassured me that I had done all that I could and he tried to restore my belief in myself as only he knew how. It was cold outside but the freshness of the air woke me up to myself and, with Jerzy's support, I was able to return again.

During the time that followed I think I was on some kind of autopilot. I turned my attention to the plans for Jess's funeral and allowed little else to dominate my mind. The care team were marvellous. The depth of care that had surrounded us all in the run-up to Jess's death now continued, with seamless experience, to encompass the whole family. Immediately after her death a silver star was placed on each of the entrances to the hospice, a sign to each member of the care team as they arrived for their shifts that a child had died. It was clear when Helen arrived that she had been very saddened by our loss and we shared that in honesty together. Arriving to see the star on the door, she had immediately known it was Jess and found this devastating. As one of our designated carers, along with Libby, she had worked closely with Jess in these previous weeks and they had become quite close. Libby and Helen now both took on a different role, one that enabled us to put together a really special funeral service for Jess. They filled in forms, took us to register her death and supported everything we felt we needed to do in order to make the service a fitting tribute to a very special child. They helped us to contact people and to find music, readings and poetry. It seemed as though everything was possible and nothing would ever be too much trouble. Little Bridge House even printed the order of service booklets with full colour pictures of Jess and the children. In their capacity to care and with their unique knowledge they were able to lift so much weight from our shoulders.

After an initial influx of people wanting to see Jess, we were left alone. I remember it felt strange in the days leading up to the funeral, as we had very limited contact with anyone unless it was something to do with the arrangements. It was as though we were sheltering from a storm beneath the huge branches of a timeless oak tree, with each leaf of that tree dedicated to protecting and preserving us as a family. In between phone calls and lists of important things to remember, I took time out and continued to sit with Jess. Still unable to spend long away from her side, I continued to read *The Lion, the Witch and the Wardrobe* out load to her as though she could still hear me and it felt important to continue. I read of Aslam's return to life following his death at the hands of the evil witch and how overjoyed the children were to see him again, beautiful, strong and true, just as he had always been. I wished the same might happen for Jess but sadly I knew it could never be, although my faith hoped and still hopes that one day our souls may be reunited.

During the week between Jess's passing and her funeral, Gemma and Stewart continued to play as they had before her death. They mixed with other siblings and we spoke with other parents. I wondered if I was passing on to them something of the gift that the little boy's mother had given to me: the knowledge that Little Bridge was a special place that they could know would be able to help them, in the same way that we were helped. They could trust in the support and honesty found there. They would know and grow from the same strength when their own time to say goodbye would come. Where else in the world but in a children's hospice would you find parents bound by the same truth? Speaking with other parents gave another dimension to the care provided there. It was about the realisation of not being alone. There was huge comfort to be found in being truly understood, and these people seemed to know our pain without the need for explanation.

The day of Jess's funeral eventually arrived and we packed and prepared to leave, knowing that we would be returning home straight afterwards. We had been supported in returning home briefly in order to look for photographs for the order of service booklet and to collect a few things. Apart from this, we had not returned home since the day we left to visit Little Bridge House for a few days in order to get Jess's symptoms under control. The development of her pneumonia had taken everyone by surprise, although her doctor had explained that it was not unusual. Her weakened immune system and declining strength gave her little reserve to fight off infection. We had been encouraged to believe that her quick decline was a blessing in many ways. The alternative would have been a long drawn-out process in which she may have suffered a great deal more. I remember reflecting on this but I still dreaded returning home. There would be a huge hole in our family now and this would be hard for everyone. Just how were we going to survive without Jess? How was I going to live without her?

I know that I confidently said goodbye and thanked everyone for their help, and I couldn't put into words how much they had helped us all, but inwardly I was a mess and dreaded today, facing people and going over it all again. I felt as though I were being forced to put on an appearance, expected to perform when all I wanted to do was to hide away in this special little world where I was safe. All I could do was go with each moment as it presented itself and do my best by Jess.

The funeral director arrived promptly along with a sea of flowers from many different people. I remember being pleased with our wreath set to adorn the top of her casket and covered in glitter. Jess was the original glitter queen and loved a bit of 'bling', so I wanted it to shine as she was carried in, representing the way she shone in the world and touched the lives of those who knew her. I had chosen a simple white casket for her, reflecting the innocence of her childhood but also the dream I'd had way back before her original diagnosis. I remembered how upset I had been to see her in a white coffin and now this vision had become truth.

We left the funeral director and his aides to move Jess from her bed into the casket and then we each spent time with her. Andrew had his time alone, then Jerzy and I. I placed a number of things in with her: a small dream catcher - she loved the notion of catching dreams and somehow I hoped her dreams had helped her through her final journey; a picture of my cousin's little boy, Aiden, who was born prematurely and remained in an incubator, but Jess was too sick to make the long journey to visit him as she had hoped; some of the flowers from Craig's bouquet and the card he had written; and a single red rose from me, the accompanying card saying, "I'll always love you, Jess. Sleep gently, my precious baby." As the lid of the casket was tightened down I was aware that I had gazed upon her face for the last time. I had continued to spend hours next to her side, having rarely been apart from her throughout her illness, but suddenly now we were finally separated and I had only my memories of our time together to hold on to.

Stewart saw her white casket being lifted into the back of the hearse and surrounded by the floral tributes that had arrived throughout the morning. He was pleased that it looked so pretty and he felt much happier and safer watching the casket than seeing her lifeless face. Gemma had dressed for the day in a bright glittery outfit and had shown little emotion during the week apart from her initial tears. I guessed today would be different and the final reality of our loss would hit home in time.

Little Bridge was at least an hour away from the church but we had arranged to travel directly there, and as this was a long journey we only slowed our speed a couple of miles from our destination. It was raining constantly, dull and grey, reflecting the mood in my heart. As we travelled I remembered the times I had travelled this road before: our initial journey, the anticipation of what we would find and my doubt that Little Bridge would be right for us. How wrong I had been about so many things and how wonderfully we had been supported through everything. I remembered the last time I had driven down, just me and the children as Jerzy was working. Jess had been in constant pain but excited to be returning for a few days in order to get her comfortable. The weather that day had been glorious, a sharp contrast to today, and she had enjoyed the spectacular views across the north Devon countryside. I was almost glad not to see the same sight today; it would've been almost too painful, as this had been our last trip and she would never return to our home again.

As we drew near the church, the roads were lined with cars but there were no people, which seemed a bit strange. I think I had expected to see people making their way through the rain towards the shelter of the church. There was a peculiar hush as I got out of the car. Only the tapping of the rain on the umbrella held over my head was apparent to me as we made our way up the path behind Jess. As I rounded the corner to go through the entrance porch my eyes met with the most beautiful tree. I suppose it had always been there seeing as Nynehead was my childhood home, but I didn't remember ever seeing it covered in blossom. Marking the entrance to the church, and through the rain, fabulous branches laden with the most beautiful white blossom were visible. It stood in stark contrast to this gloomy wet day, the only tree I had witnessed in bloom that early this spring. Its presence left a deep impression on me. It seemed as though it bloomed for Jess, Mother Nature acknowledging

171

Jess's love of all things and making her presence known for this special little girl.

Entering the church was again another surprise to me, as it was completely filled with people. There were faces everywhere and people standing wherever they could, clearly wanting to be involved in remembering Jess. For the last week we had been cocooned in the quiet safety of Little Bridge, surrounded and knowing our own grief. I had guessed there would be a lot of people who would want to attend her funeral but the numbers that packed this tiny village church that day were a huge shock to me. Sad eyes reflected the glow of the hundreds of candles flickering around the church as Jess was carried gently down the aisle with the song she had sung with Myleene Klass playing in the background. She was placed behind the ornately carved screen in front of the altar, where I had sat as a member of the church choir at the same age as Jess. There were flowers displayed on every available shelf, complementing the candles which even floated in the open font. There were lilac, silver and ivory balloons arranged in tasteful displays arching over the aisle that Jess had passed along. It was a truly beautiful setting and it was filled with the loving warmth of so many family and friends. Most importantly to me, there were children there - something that I had tried to encourage, hoping that their parents would give them the chance to say goodbye to their own special friend. At a certain point in the service the children from the primary school placed posies of flowers they had made around a central candle. Jess would have been so proud to see them all there. It was just as she had wanted when she had spoken briefly of her funeral wishes.

It was a fabulous service and a true celebration of a beautiful child who gave so much to so many. I was then, and will always be, so proud of her and so proud to have been her mum. Many of the staff from the hospice were there: they had prepared and managed the music, they took photographs of the church to help me remember, and they continued to support our needs on this most difficult of days. How could I have managed so well without them - surely angels in disguise? Rain hammered down as we left the church and Jess was placed into the hearse once more, this time making a final journey to the crematorium. I chatted for a while, sheltered by a huge black umbrella, and when I was finally urged to get into the car I was shivering with the cold and wet through. As we drove I remembered how this was Jess's express wish, although I dreaded it with every ounce of my being. I had wanted to bury her precious form, so that it would be safely resting in the churchyard I had known since childhood. However, Jess had expressed a wish to be cremated. She wanted the cancer burnt from her body and who was I to deny her final wish. As we arrived I felt sick and I could barely place one foot in front of the other as we followed Jess's casket for the final time. Jerzy and Sarah supported me on either side and guided me towards the front. This had been intended for close family only, a final intimate farewell, but again there was an unexpected gathering of people. No service had been planned this time; our celebration of this treasured life was over. This was the final committal of her body for cremation; a sad, stark few moments of painful reality, and a huge contrast to the warmth of the church. I had wanted this to be as short as possible and it was. I had not expected so many to attend as we had encouraged people to wait for us at the village hall where refreshments had been arranged. Leaving her there was the hardest single thing I have ever done. My dearest, darling Jess, my precious baby and my friend. My loss was overwhelming.

I was helped back to the car, too cold and shocked to stand in the rain once more and greet people. I remember feeling embarrassed by the rawness of my emotions being on public display. People could still see me through the windows of the car as they left the building. I just wanted to be on my own. I felt as though I couldn't breathe.

The driver put the heaters on in the car and soon we were on our way back to the hall to join my younger children. I have never felt pain like it; it was as though someone had ripped a piece of my very soul away, leaving me squirming and gasping for air. By the time we arrived at the hall I had managed to compose myself a bit. I know that I talked to a lot of people, one after another, and I remember some faces, but mostly the memory of this time is a blur to me. I know that the team from the hospital were there and, of course, Nicky: the warm, friendly faces of those who had cared for Jess continuously for the longest time, from the beginning of our journey, and now here they were at the end. I am so very grateful to them all for their dedication and commitment to Jess's needs. I know that we moved on to being welcomed by Little Bridge, but we never forgot those who had travelled as far as they could with us. I remember moving around, trying to be friendly and sociable. Autopilot had kicked in again. I expect I repeated myself a lot, saying what I felt was right at the time. I think I continued to look for reassurance that I had done and said the right things, but I was no longer held solely within the extraordinary environment that was Little Bridge House. These dear friends and family could never know or completely understand our journey in the same way as the care team and other families who had shared the same pain. Retrospectively I think I was in shock at suddenly finding myself amongst so many people after having kept a graceful, peaceful space at the hospice for a number of weeks, but particularly following Jess's death. I felt alone, suddenly without Jess's physical presence next to me, that closeness that typified our relationship. I remember Gemma and Stewart running around with other children from the village and they enjoyed meeting with their friends again. Somehow children are so much more able than adults to bounce in and out of pain. Jess's siblings had no doubt found the day hard but they moved on quickly in this space, returning to play with a familiar sense of fun and blissfully unaware of their mother's struggling soul.

Eventually there were just a few of us left tidying up, and I was encouraged to sit down for the first time with a cup of tea. Jerzy suddenly realised that we had not made arrangements to get home from the hall, so a few willing volunteers rallied together to give us all a lift home, including our luggage, enabling us finally to retreat to our own space once more. As we piled out of various cars Gemma ran up our shared driveway, trailing a string of helium balloons from the church and coloured as a sparkly rainbow. She was met by our new neighbour who had moved in whilst we were all away.

She greeted Gemma enthusiastically. "Hello, have you just been to a party?"

To which Gemma innocently replied, "No, my sister's

funeral."

I'm sure her heart must have sunk when she realised her mistake, but we explained as quickly as possible and it became a well-remembered beginning to a good friendship.

The following day the rain retreated and the sun broke through as we made our way solemnly to the church once more, this time to commit Jess's ashes to the ground in the company of a few close friends and family. Her grave had already been prepared when we arrived: a small hole in the ground surrounded by the children's flowers from the day before. Andrew and his family were there along with other close friends and of course Sarah and her children. The true splendour of my tree could really be appreciated today. The blossom appeared crisp and fresh in this new sunlight. I remembered how the whiteness of the blooms had stood out in sharp contrast against the grey wet day that had gone before. The memory of this tree sits poignantly in my mind. I will never forget the presence it had as we gently laid this small wooden casket to rest in the shadow of its branches. Andrew stood for a while with his arm around me, a chance to reflect on our shared loss and a moment I appreciated greatly. I felt able to breathe today. I had a clearer head and was more settled in myself. I felt that Jess was now at home, resting in the churchyard she knew so well and in the shade of the most beautiful white tree.

Chapter 17

In the strongest sense, following Jess's death I felt overwhelmed by the desire to make a difference somehow. I wanted her life to count for something and found it hard to accept the pointlessness of her passing. How could this happen unless for some greater purpose? I needed to find a reason. After spending so much of my days focusing on caring for Jess, there was a huge void in my life now, one that I started to fill with activities surrounding fund-raising, public speaking at sometimes quite large events and involvement in raising awareness for improved palliative care services for children. I would tell Jess's story to anyone prepared to listen, in the hope that something of what I had to say might make a difference. In making that difference I would find my reason for Jess having given her life in the way she did. However, at a personal level, I wasn't coping. I would have denied it then, but I now know it was true. Grief overwhelmed me and it was hard to hide the rawness of that emotion, which ebbed and flowed. Sometimes I would manage to hide what was going on for me, and then something would happen and complete devastation would wash over me again like a huge wave, relentless in momentum. I would drown in such dark sorrow. It was as though I had travelled to the edge of dying myself in order to remain by her side, in order to keep my promise and always be there for her. At the point that she left me, I felt that a part of my soul went away too, leaving only a shadow of my former self behind. Then began the long, dark and sometimes lonely trek home. I have no doubt that a combination of my public activities and a deep-seated instinct to continue to be a mother and a wife kept me going - strong, loving relationships that nourished me and provided a reason to survive.

The care team at Little Bridge House, Helen and Libby in particular, kept in touch and carried on the caring concern that became a guiding light in my darkness. They would telephone every so often and I could contact them whenever I needed to, always finding comfort in sharing my experience with people who just knew how it was for us. They would come and visit as well and share a cup of tea or join in with some of the events we organised. We never seem to be forgotten, and returning for 'Remembering Day' every year has become a real focal point in our family's calendar: a time when we meet up with old friends, sharing memories and experiences. There is not only a sharing of intense sadness but also there is happiness in the warmth of family friendship and shared joy. This is a special place where treasured memories are fashioned. Love and laughter survive in the hearts of these families even though they have all experienced unimaginable sadness.

Gemma and Stewart also meet with other siblings, enjoy playing around the house and remember Jess in their own ways. In the afternoon there is a service of remembrance when parents and siblings are invited to join in with poems, songs and stories that have special meaning to their own families. This takes place in a spacious marquee decorated with pictures of the children who have died, along with flowers and plants. There is usually a water feature, providing a gentle, comforting trickle in the background, surrounded by a carefully fashioned sand pool. During the service families are invited to light candles and place them in the sand where they are left to burn through the afternoon. It is a moving and very special shared experience; a reflection of the sadness that binds us all but also giving rise to the sense of not being alone.

At the hospice our loss is always acknowledged and accepted. There is no judgement or expectation of how long the process will take. When we arrive it is like stepping off onto another dimension where time and expectation have no meaning and everything is simply just the way it is. It is a healing space, a place to recognise and be free to express how we feel and to learn to move forward gently. Immediately after we lost Jess we were surrounded by people wishing us well, deeply saddened by our experience and their own felt loss. As time went by so life went on, and people naturally withdrew in order to continue with their lives. The relentless nature of our world is to continue turning, doing, busying and growing, completely unaware of how another's world can stand still. I watched Jess's friends from a distance growing up. I would see them walking along the side of the road on their way home from school, happy in their thoughts, playful and carefree. I would mark time by birthdays, Christmases and anniversaries, with all sorts of questions in my head. What might she be like now? How would she have changed? Would I recognise her or the sound of her voice? My experience stayed with me; this was my world, as though I stood still and everybody and everything else rushed by. At Little Bridge House this was understood as a difficulty faced by all parents: the need to still validate the lost relationship and to keep alive the memory of that precious life. I have come to recognise that Jess is a part of me, she always will be, and I hold her essence in my heart. I wonder if, just as a part of me went with her, perhaps a piece of her rests within me, maybe giving me the strength to have changed direction so drastically and now be working to support the emotional needs of others.

Immediately following Jess's death, a number of things happened that held a particular importance to me and that I now consider as special experiences that go beyond coincidence or synchronicity. My first was a dream like no other I have ever had before or have experienced since. It was not unusual for me during my saddest moments to find myself in a kind of half-conscious sleep; a place where I still experienced my grief and my body was not quite given to complete rest. I remember that my eyes were closed. This did not happen against the backdrop of my room, there was darkness all around. Jess appeared before me. Her hair had grown long and was swept back from her face by a gentle breeze. Her face was glowing with a radiant complexion and she smiled with such joyous excitement. She was so real to me that I felt I could have reached out and touched her. In my wonder I smiled back, and although unable to reach her maybe our joy met somewhere in the space between us. I asked her questions and this is how I know I was quite conscious, because I remember choosing what to say with great care.

"Are you all right?"

She glanced sideways as though she were receiving guidance and then nodded excitedly back at me.

"What's it like, Jess?"

She glanced away again and then smiled back sensitively.

"You can't tell me, can you?"

Without glancing away this time, she shook her head.

"I'll always love you, Jess, my special angel. Keep safe and maybe we'll be together again some day."

As she smiled, her dimple clearly visible, I felt touched by her love for me.

"Thank you, Jess."

Then she was gone. There was darkness all around but I felt I had been blessed by her presence.

A few days later Jerzy and I were on our way to pick up some photographs when we paused to look in a shop window. Suddenly the shopkeeper came out and said he had something he felt he wanted to show us. This seemed a bit strange; the kind of behaviour you might expect in some European marketplaces but not something I had ever experienced in Taunton high street. Curiosity got the better of us and we followed him in. He took us to a stand in the centre of the shop where glass ornaments were displayed. He picked up the largest in the centre and gave it to me. It was a solid piece of glass with a finely shaped, domed top. Suspended in the centre was the image of an angel playing a stringed instrument and surrounded by flowers, laser etched in fine, exquisite detail, capturing a sense of peace and serenity as she floated tenderly in this sensitive space. Neither of us really knew what to say. I felt as though this was a symbol for us both, a message of some kind. I felt that Jess had found her peace and wanted us to know through the touch of this angel. Angels had come to hold a deeper level of significance for me through my discussions about heaven with Jess. I had told her that she would be the brightest angel in heaven, and knowing this made the experience of this glass angel all the more special. In the months that followed I also felt driven to painting angels, beautiful images of light and serenity, images painted in a way that I had never explored before. Although artistic in my abilities, these paintings were out of character for me and a complete surprise. They represented the honesty of the visions I had created with words to Jess: the gentleness, the colour, the warmth and the peace. Four particular images were published as prints and greetings cards. I wasn't particularly successful at selling them, but I gave them away to various charity events and Gemma sold them at school for various fund-raising activities. Sometimes I gave them away to people I felt would benefit from them and occasionally I received e-mails or letters from people who felt helped in some way. This type of feedback was special and gave the paintings relevance and meaning. But they never were just pictures or cards to me. These angels held a profound significance; they were a special connection with Jess that I didn't completely understand. Sometimes it's better to accept 'what is' rather than try to understand it. These angels were spontaneous and beautiful, a reflection of something really special to both Jess and me. Curiously, once these four images were completed I never painted any more angels.

There have been countless occasions when music has touched me in some way. There is nothing unusual about that because music has the potential to impact us all and particular songs hold individual meaning for every one of us. Jess and I had often sung together, having our very favourite songs which lightened our mood and allowed moments of real joy to surface between us. Sometimes singing together enabled true connection where words were not appropriate but the gentleness of a shared song said it all. She understood our connection through music and presented this quite powerfully when we shared our last moments in the jacuzzi together at Little Bridge House. She had been in intense pain but wanted to remain in our gentle, peaceful space together until the Eva Cassidy CD, she had bought me for Christmas, had finished. She had known how those words touched me and had been determined to share that time. In those painful months that followed her passing, apart from missing her intensely, I would often struggle with whether I had done enough and had I made the right decisions for Jess when she was no longer able to voice her own feelings? In my deepest, darkest moments I often found I would hear, quite randomly, a familliar song playing in the background or whilst walking through a shopping centre, for instance, a street musician bringing to life once more the words and music which Jess knew touched me deeply. I felt she was offering me reassurance and continuing to reach out to me. These instances would happen so frequently they came not to be a surprise anymore but special moments of continued connection which meant the world to me. Objectively, of course, these can be regarded simply as insignificant happenings that can be explained away as nothing at all. Maybe this bereaved parent wanted to see and hear things of significance, but to me there seems no harm in believing that we don't have all the answers. No one can say for sure what happens after we die and therefore I prefer to believe that we continue in some way.

I would often have a sense of Jess standing alongside me. I made the children laugh one day when I bought five doughnuts from the bakers and had a real sense of walking home in the company of three children. Perhaps it was similar to the sensation that people have when a limb is amputated - phantom pains and a sense of the limb still existing. When I stand up to speak in public I also have this same feeling, as though she is stood by the side of me giving me the strength to say what needs to be said. It's a special experience, as though I can almost see her in the very periphery of my vision, encouraging something good to come out of our sadness.

It was this desire to make a difference somehow that was the driving force behind my returning to college. This was the beginning of a different journey, a complete change in direction and a reassessment of my own personal awareness and ability. Working towards becoming a counsellor has felt a courageous pathway requiring commitment to self-development and working through painful elements of life experience. I now help individuals to come to terms with their own psychological pain and to find a sense of peace and direction in their lives. My experience changed me to a point where I am now able to sit in complete empathy with others in the depths of intense sadness, to walk alongside them, gently helping them find their own way towards a more positive future.

About a year after Jess died we returned to the hospice for a special weekend, a time when we took part in activities together surrounding loss. We met with other families and the parents were accommodated in a nearby hotel while the children all stayed together at Little Bridge. Gemma and Stewart joined in with making photo frames, mobiles and pictures. They used things collected from the beach, colourful papers, feathers, sequins and, of course, glue and paint. Stewart really treasured his 'memory stones', which he put together over this weekend: a shiny stone for special memories, a pretty stone for good times and a rough stone for the horrible memories. They were tied up in a piece of cloth on which he drew some pictures of individual importance to him. He still keeps these precious stones today. We did a balloon release together, sending words on the wind to our children, and we also took part in activities that bound us together as people with similar shared loss, emphasising the sense of family that is echoed throughout Little Bridge. The children went on trips out with the other siblings and one evening, to Gemma and Stewart's delight, they went to the nearby pub for supper and a game of skittles. Then at dusk they went down to the estuary and released paper boats carrying candles and watched as they drifted gently away. This was a poignant and moving moment for them both, one that they often mentioned afterwards with a deep sense of respect and understanding. As they each told me about this, I imagined all the children joined together in a quiet sharing of this profound moment of remembrance, the gentle stillness of the evening water and the reflections of the candlelight drifting peacefully out of sight.

Both Gemma and Stewart managed well overall. I know there have been times when individually they have found their loss hard to carry, but they have both continued in life with courage. Honesty has continued to be at the core of our journey together and has given them each a solid foundation from which to grow. It wasn't always easy to understand their reactions, but children are better than adults at going with the moment and reflecting in all innocence just how it is for them. For instance, Gemma's initial reaction was to be sometimes quite joyous - hard to accept when sorrow may have seemed more appropriate. But in Gemma's world she was pleased: there would be no more despair surrounding caring for Jess, no more terrifying hallucinations in the night, no more strangers in our house at all hours. She would not bear witness to Jess's suffering anymore. She visualised her sister as now being free, and with that notion came a genuine sense of joy. She did cry, however, and she would choose to speak to trusted friends particularly at school.

I think, in a way, she tried to protect me from her sadness. She rarely shared her thoughts with me, but so long as she was talking to someone, whoever that might be, I knew that she would be okay.

In the early days I worried about her tummy aches, which I often had checked out and sought medical opinions on. I had lost all sense of what was 'normal' for not feeling well. I was constantly concerned that it may be something worse, as it had been for poor Jess. I had never been told 'why', and in all honesty I don't think anybody ever knew. But this left me feeling as though whatever had caused Jess's cancer may also have affected Gemma and Stewart. It was a genuine fear that haunted me for a long time, and each time one of them was feeling under the weather I would go into panic mode. Needless to say, they were both fine and healthy and in time my fears subsided. I understood how rare her illness was and that the chances of her siblings developing the same cancer were extremely remote.

Gradually Gemma has grown in confidence and has enjoyed her many sporting passions, including trampolining, which at one time took up a fair-sized chunk of every week. She has loved school, making many genuine friendships which she truly values. At the time of finishing this book she is attending a drama school in Exeter where she has been developing her singing, dancing and acting skills. For a few years we joined the Amateur Dramatic Association at Nynehead and took part, as a family, in the annual pantomime. This was a fabulous family activity and gave us a chance to think about something new together, and Gemma's love for drama undoubtedly grew from here. When I watch her performing now I am moved beyond words to see her developing such potential. She has tremendous presence, tall and elegant. She also has a special kind of grace about her, which may well have been influenced by her experience. It is almost certainly a quality that cannot be learned but comes from somewhere special within. With all she has been through, she has done so well and I am proud to be able to support her dreams. I know that whatever pathway she chooses the determination and free spirit that have always flowed through Gemma in abundance will continue to carry her courageously into the future.

When Stewart was born Jess was four years old. She loved having a baby brother and helped bath him, change him and cuddle him at every opportunity. She took the responsibility of being a 'big sister' very seriously and became like a little mummy to him. There was a lot of sisterly rivalry between Gemma and Jess, as might be expected, but Stewart sat outside this healthy competition and was never in demand of her clothes, make-up or toys in the same way as Gemma. To understand the dynamic between the three of them was to understand how losing Jess affected poor Stewie. Jess had always been there, watching over him, loving him and caring for him. When he first went to school she promised to take care of him at playtime, always watchful of his needs and wary of his vulnerability. Communication was difficult for him and he had struggled to learn. It was clear from an early age that he learned in different ways to the girls and school was always going to be an uphill task. When Jess died it was as though his world imploded on him. He spent much of his time alone at play and in silence. He would be obsessive about tasks, becoming completely engrossed, as though in a different world or in his own dimension. It took a long time for us to be able to reach him and for him to find a way out of the place into which he retreated. Trying to get him extra help at school was hard initially, as it was difficult for the professionals to identify where he was experiencing genuine problems with learning and separate those from the results of grieving. The teaching staff at Nynehead Primary School were incredibly understanding, supportive and helpful, but in order to give weight to his need for extra assistance we took Stewart to BIBIC (The British Institute for Brain Injured Children). They ran a series of tests on him over a few days and were able to help us to help him. We learned how we could help him to learn, how he received information, the things that were helpful and those that were not. We also looked at his diet, changing to healthier alternatives and keeping him away from chocolate and anything containing food additives. He was given a programme of tasks to complete every day, exercises that were aimed at improving his balance and fine motor skills in order to enhance the way his brain sent messages from one side to the other. There were also physical activities that worked specifically on his retained reflexes. The combination of the changes we made as a result and the honesty we shared as a family enabled Stewart quite suddenly to begin to flourish. He really came to enjoy school and related well to the friends he had around him. He developed a wicked sense of humour and loved to tease, although I remember clearly the day he told his headmistress she was having 'a bad hair day'! Stewart has gone from strength to strength, achieving well at school and actively developing his sporting ability. I am so proud of his confidence; when I think of how hard it was for him to find it, he has done so well. Just like all boys of his age he loves the latest gaming technology, spending hours finding his way through the most complex of games. He has also developed a keen artistic eye and produces fabulous drawings of intricate detail. He is a joy to be around; a loving, considerate child who has travelled his own difficult journey and who, just like his sister, is now striving for his future with tremendous commitment and courage.

And so, as a family, we have found a way forward and the world no longer passes us by. Gradually we have grown together as a new family, a family of four instead of five. Honesty has been a guiding light in my darkest moments. Even Jess thanked me for my honesty and said she was glad that she knew what was happening to her. She said that she would have felt betrayed had I not been so honest and I am so glad that we never went down that path. My advice to all parents would be always to hold a sense of honesty with your children. They are stronger than they may seem and often instinctively know when something is going on. It's better to be honest than to leave them making up their own sense of reality and feeling alone. A combination of time and the professional training I have embarked on has enabled me to carry a sense of Jess with me and I no longer feel overwhelmed by loss. I feel as though I am living again, achieving so much for myself and for other people too. As a bodily response to the intensity of my experience I developed arthritis, which has taken several years to diminish in power, and I am so pleased it finally has. Part of my development as a counsellor has been to recognise the way in which our bodies are so connected to our emotional experience.

When there is emotional pain it is often manifested as physical pain, and understanding what that pain is about can be the key to finding a sense of well being again.

Together we developed ways of remembering Jess. Apart from the activities we shared at Little Bridge we did our own special and meaningful things, which kept a sense of Jess as remaining a part of our family. Just as Stewart had said he wanted to, we lit candles at mealtimes and on special occasions. We painted the house yellow, just as Jess had wanted us to. We put collages of photographs on the walls, including pictures of the children at all ages. Over the years since Jess left us I have put together several new ones, but I always include pictures of her to show that she is still held within the heart of our family. We often mention her name and remember her in our conversations; she is a part of our daily lives and always will be. I remember one time we made a kite together and Stewart taped a photo of Jess to it. We took it to the playing field adjacent to the church at Nynehead. It was a very gusty day and the kite lifted effortlessly into the air. I felt we were setting her free as her picture rose high in the sky. When I turned around I could see Jess's grave nestled against the perimeter wall of the graveyard and sheltered under my special tree. Its branches were swirling in the hearty breeze as though waving at us all with joy.

I often visited Jess's grave, particularly when Gemma and Stewart were still at school. I planted it out in the shape of a heart and decorated it with fairies, animals, butterflies and dragonflies. It became a tiny garden of remembrance where we could place things collected from the beach or brought back from holidays. We could light candles on birthdays and decorate it at Christmas. On a good day I could sit on the grass alongside in quiet reflection. Sometimes I would talk as though she were there, or just tend to the plants and drink in the tranquillity of this tiny corner of countryside. I would be able to hear the chattering laughter of the children in the nearby school playground, where Jess had played and known such happiness. Always I was aware of my tree, standing firm by my shoulder, rustling in the wind as I whispered a quiet prayer. No one I knew was able to name this tree and yet everyone remarked on its beauty, particularly when in bloom. It occurred to me that this tree had been quietly present for the whole of my lifetime. It had heard me playing in the playground. I had passed beneath its branches as a baby being christened and attending church as a growing child. This tree had witnessed me as a bride and then as a mother of three beautiful children of my own. Then she had experienced my sadness, perhaps as a Mother in Nature herself, and she had seen my tears and sheltered me from the rain as I had openly grieved. Always standing quietly in the corner, magnificent and yet unnoticed and rarely appreciated, it occurred to me that she was a guardian, a silent companion in my life and now watching over my precious child. She lays her leaves like a blanket in winter to comfort and protect. She shakes her blossom like mighty white wings to hail the beginning of spring. Her white petals fall gently to the ground as confetti at a wedding. In summer there is cool, refreshing shade and a gentle, musical rustle as the breeze flows through her branches. This tree has a special name, she is my Angel Tree.

As I sit here beneath my Angel Tree with the sun on my face and surrounded by tranquillity, I am aware of the immense journey that we have travelled as a family; of the changes I have made and my new-found commitment to bettering the lives of others who are suffering emotional sadness. I believe that I have found my purpose and I believe that Jess is a huge part of my newly discovered abilities; she is my inspiration and always will be. In terms of making a difference, I know that Jess did that, and her story has touched the hearts of many. Her strength and courage have changed lives, with people following different pathways, raising money and working to assist other families who wrestle with the same difficulties that we did. I'm sure, too, that professional learning has resulted from her treatment and that the samples taken from her liver have informed science, hopefully helping to develop a better understanding of childhood cancers. Our experience went towards spurring the development of a new Children's Community Palliative Care Service, providing support for local families. The money we personally helped to raise went in two directions: towards building the new hospice, Charlton Farm near Bristol, and also upgrading the accommodation on the children's ward in

Musgrove Park Hospital.

In October 2003, Myleene Klass launched her debut album *Moving On* which she dedicated to Jessica. Myleene wrote "A special dedication to Jessica Leigh-Firbank and her family - an amazing young lady that I was lucky enough to meet and play the piano with. She is now 'home again' but always in our hearts". Myleene had clearly been deeply touched by their meeting and Jess would have been so proud of that.

About a year after Jess died I visited a lady who professed to be able to hear spirits and she told me that I was writing a book, which I was, and that Jess had told her to tell me, "a book's not a book until it's finished". She also said that many people would read this book and it would help more people than I might ever realise. Well Jess, I am now finished. It has taken over five years and has not been easy at all. Writing has undoubtedly helped me find direction, though, mapping my way home and towards a more settled future with Jerzy, Gemma and Stewart. It has been an enormous journey through which you taught me so much and I know you would be very proud that your story will be benefitting other children and their families that follow. I truely hope there is a chance your strength and courage will continue to reach out to people through the pages of this book and make a difference somehow, like the branches of a tree reaching towards the sunlight, providing both shade and comfort to those in need.

As I make my way down the pathway towards the wrought-iron church gate, there are beams of sunlight filtering through the huge chestnut trees. I smile to myself as I remember all those who have cared for Jess and our whole family: pictures and faces; caring, understanding and supportive faces accompanied by extraordinary memories and experiences for which no parent could ever be prepared. I thank you all and I know that Jess would thank you too. I also thank my dear husband for being the rock beneath my feet, for his loving encouragement, but mostly for believing in me. For Gemma and Stewart, my two beautiful children, I love and thank you both for being so uniquely special and a complete joy in my life. Jess, I am so proud to have been your mum and privileged to have learned so much from you. I will carry you in my heart always and pray that one day we may be reunited. My one regret remains that I was unable to find a way through my grief in time to save my relationship with Sarah. I miss her and the girls in my life and so wish that things could have worked out differently.

And finally, in glancing back I see once more my tree, silently strong above my daughter's grave. I don't feel the need to return so often now as I know my dear Jess rests in peace. The memories of our love and her radiant smile will live in my heart always. I know that my silent guardian in life now watches over her, tender branches reaching towards the sunlight, providing both shade and comfort to those in need, just as she did for me: my Angel Tree.

Tributes & Memories

Our joys will be greater
Our love will be deeper
Our life will be fuller
Because we shared your moment
- (Unknown)

Dear God
Please look after Jessica very well in heaven
Help her family when they are sad
Jessica was very nice and we all miss her very much.
- Amen from Kate

Jess was the best
Better than anyone
Always helpful, always kind
Loving and Caring, one of a kind

Pets she adored
Especially hers
Snowy the Rabbit
Along with Ginger Geri
Who was small and merry

Fashion she knew a lot about
Designer jeans with a sparkly top
She wore these things a lot
Pilot was her favourite shop
Always came up at the top

I miss Jess like a dog with a bone
I always think of her when at home
I remember her in my thoughts
Thank you Jess, for lots & lots!
- Love from Becky

Jessica was my best friend. We played together.
We made Halloween costumes. We went to the beach.
We took Jet to the monument and played on the old cannon.
We went down a steep hill. She was very kind and helpful.
I will miss Jessica's lovely voice.
- By Hayley

My Little Cousin Jess
Maybe it's the mist of time, or maybe this was true,
But Jess you were a happy child, you smiled lots as you grew,
We miss you Jess, we do

I remember you as a toddler, you loved to entertain
To have a captive audience, was hours of endless games,
You were always seeking company, always being a friend,
You loved to make us laugh Jess, this gift just grew no end.
We miss you Jess, we do

You always had a tale to tell, a joke or silly game,
No matter how tired or sad you were,
You'd find the irony all the same!
How you loved to entertain
We miss you Jess, we do

I learnt from you Jess, not to shy away
You loved your God and trusted him, and lent on him always
When life hurts I think of you
"What would Jess say?" I muse
I know you'd tell me to smile and be..
Exactly what God has created in me.

I'm saddened that it took your life,
So wise and Eleven years
To open my eyes to living – but Jess,
I'm grateful, despite my tears.

I will never forget your laugh and humour,
I am inspired to be like you.
To smile at what life throws at me,
And grasp each day, anew.

I miss you Jess, I do
- Rest in peace, Love Bizzy

Life is a Gift
Jess you were a breath in time,
A mere whisper in 'times' conversation
Just as we were knowing you,
Eternity took you home

We feel cheated now, it seems unjust,
To glimpse the wonderful person of Jess,
Yet asked to give her back, no less.
Memories, forever Memories.

I trust you are at peace Jess, I know my God and yours.
Is it really what is promised, truly awesome to behold?
Have you found some friends Jess?
Have you forgotten pain and fear?

Are your eyes sparkling bright again?
We long to hold you near.
We'd give anything to change this, to selfishly have you home,
But God had other plans for you, and you'll never be alone.
- Love always Bizzy

I remember when I very first met Jessica, she'd been attending a school in Milverton and was looking to move to our school. I got to show her around and a friendship established immediately. That September she started and that was the start of the best friendship I've ever had. My memories from our days at primary school are so important to me, and are so different to what many other people have from their primary school. As our school was only small, holding only one class, me and Jess managed to spend the majority of our lessons, play times and lunches together. Soon without realising we became inseparable. The main things we used to do in primary school were dance, laugh and sit in the round house, something we made together as part of a team.

If there was one thing I had to say thanks to Jess for then its making me smile. Jess was the girl at school that was compatible with everyone, helpful and outgoing – an enlightenment to be around, a pleasure to be near and an amazing best friend. Jess and I had a unique friendship, she'd do anything for me and I would for her. I only remember falling out with Jess the once, we walked to the petrol station to get some sweets and I left her brand new furby down there ~ we walked back down, found the furby and got more sweets! Jess just laughed it off. I also *remember trick or treating with jess one Halloween, we dressed up and to our horror looked more like clowns, but still set off. We laughed and screamed the whole way round, then went back to Jess's and told horror stories until it was time for me to go. Looking back me and jess spent the most time we possibly could together. During the summer holidays we'd walk with the family to the river to play 'poo sticks'. We'd play in the park, go swimming and have sleepovers.*

In the September when I became a year 6, we were the closest we'd ever been. We talked all day at school and I'd occasionally ring her once I'd got home. We spent a lot of time together. As the months past by and the SAT's were over, I had come to the time when I had to go to secondary school, it was so hard. I'd had such a great time and made a good bunch of friends and had a solid best friend. I didn't want to leave. September of that year I started Kingsmead, which meant seeing a lot less of Jess. However we made the most of the opportunities we had and met at the weekends. It was shortly after leaving my best friend that I phoned every night, I'd get home and be straight on the phone. We'd speak about how we were, that day at school, friends, teachers and the weekend ahead. Jess would talk to me about my problems and I did the same for her and even more we'd always make each other laugh and smile. I recall at one point during our phone calls, Jess said she wasn't feeling too great. She'd had trouble breathing and felt constantly ill. Jess had stopped attending school from that point, but she tried to attend school as often as she could. As of then there was less frequency in our communication and any we had was brief. I'm not sure what happened from then, which is sad, but as an 11 – 12 year old girl I didn't know what cancer entailed – other than that Jess was seriously ill.

Mum kept me on the straight and narrow reminding me that I had to be there for Jess, keeping her spirits up as she would have done for me. When Jess started going into hospital it was hard, I couldn't just call or see her. The constant thought on my mind made my school work fall behind. Mum would take me over to see Jess in hospital as often as possible and I would sit with her for as long as I could. Somehow, even while Jess was in hospital she always found the best in everything. I went in once, she was laughing so hard about The Vicar of Dibley, the video's that Kirsty had taken in for her. She was talking to me about her chemotherapy and showing me her 'Wigglies', Mr. Mrs. and Baby. (the nicknames for the three ends of her hickman line) I don't think anyone could have kept their spirit like she kept hers.

From here things got harder and harder, Jess went to bigger hospitals for better treatment and care. There were fewer times that I got to see or talk to Jess, she would ring me from her ward. She'd tell me about her operations, the nurses and on a lighter note about 'Steps' and 'Hearsay', her two favourite bands. Jess gave me a signed picture from when she went to see Hearsay. Jess was always thoughtful and sharing.

I came home from school one night; mum sat me down and said that I was going to see jess on Saturday. She said I needed to have a good chat with her, as she was starting to feel down, she had lost her hair and the chemotherapy was making her blue. It was only then mum had told me that the family had been staying in a specialist hospice to support them and prepare them, in the event of the worst. I couldn't help but cry. I was scared that my best friend wouldn't want to see me and even more I was scared that I was going to lose her. Jess had been there for me so much and I couldn't let that go – I didn't want to. I met with Jess and the family that Saturday. At first Jess was tense, quiet and unrelaxed, but she gave in and we started chatting. We spoke for hours before heading into town to do some shopping and for tea at KFC. Every action we took that day meant the world to me. Jess had never once shown or even told me of her fear until that day. Jess told me that day how she appreciated having such a wonderful family, for friends like me and told me how scared she was for her future. I had to stay strong. For Jess. When I got home after KFC, I cried. I never thought once during the day that it would be the last time

I saw my best friend.

The weeks passed ever so slowly from then, mum heard more from Kirsty than I did from Jess. My birthday was nearing and all I could do was pray that Jess would be there. I held tight to every twinge of hope until a few days before Kirsty rang to say there's little chance. My brother got a card through the post from Jess for Valentine's Day and he sent her flowers. At the same time a card came through the post for my birthday but I knew not to open it yet, my birthday was only a week away. It was the day before my birthday, February 18th, that the worst happened, I wasn't told until the 19th, but Kirsty had been trying to call. It was about 7am that mum came into my room, she woke me and I could immediately tell she was crying. Her words, 'I'm sorry', said it all. She explained that Kirsty had called and explained that jess lost the fight on the 18th. I believe she never gave up though.

I opened the card on my birthday and I could see that Jess was still trying to fight it. There were a ring of tiny little star shapes in the card and within them she wrote, with one letter in each star - 'sorry I won't be there for your birthday'. The effort she put in to getting it right was touching. That's the way I will always remember Jess. I was heartbroken. I couldn't imagine her not being there any more, not talking to her or seeing her again. The weirdest thing was that I still picked the phone up, even when I was hurting that much from her going. It is only when something like that happens that you realise what you had. Jess was so important in my life. From the day I met her, she grew from my friend to my sister and nothing will ever take that from me.

If I had to say one last thing to Jess, one last letter or one last call it would speak as follows;

You're the best friend I have always had and always will. You made me smile and glorified my laugh and above all of that you're my role model. I found love for you, for who you are and I will feel that no matter where you are.

I love you and miss you so, so much.

- Best friends – always and forever,
Kylie

I know this is short as there is so much that I could write here. The main thing I have to say is 'Thank you Jess'. We had a very unique friendship that means a lot to me, and I miss it so much. I am so lucky to have been friends with Jess, she was very influential in my childhood and I truly owe her a big thanks.

- I miss you, always in my heart. Love - Craig

On the wall of the Education Unit's portakabin, there is an art gallery of student's work.

Last week, someone asked, "Who did that painting of an eagle? It's brilliant"

I replied that it was one of many pieces of outstanding work done by Jessie, who died earlier this year after fighting very hard against cancer. I then suggested that he might like to read the Gazette Newspaper cutting about Jessie that was pasted on the cupboard door.

I told him that Jessie had a lot in common with the eagle that she chose to draw. She was a high flyer – talented in so many ways and would have undoubtedly been able to take her pick of university courses.

Like the eagle, Jessie was strong and a fighter. She never gave up her battle against the cancer and remained positive throughout the surgery and unpleasant medical procedures that she endured. She had poise and beauty, an inner confidence nurtured by her close and loving family.

If you ask someone if they have ever seen an eagle, I have no doubt they could give you the exact location and the date. It is a rare event that you remember and treasure, something out of the ordinary that can lift your spirits.

"You must miss her, "said my student.
"Yes, I do. We all do"
- Jenny Fisher, Teacher
Children's Education Unit, Musgrove Park Hospital

A routine phone call in January 2001 from Somerset Education at
County Hall introduced me to Jessie; "Would I like to teach Jessica
Leigh-Firbank, Year 6 age ten?" She was just coming out of hospital,
after investigation and treatment for cancer. She was not the first cancer
patient whom I had taught, but she was the first with liver cancer. Would
she be able to follow in the others' footsteps, cheerfully shaving the
remains of her hair after the ravages of chemotherapy, don a hat and get
back to study alongside all her friends in school?" And only ten years old,
probably without the spirit of independence which the teens bring and yet
with so much to face...Such were my thoughts as I drove through
Nynehead.

I never plan to teach much the first time I meet pupils – this is vital
time for them to say how they feel about study, what they are interested
in, what they can cope with...then I can plan round them. I found a
positivie smiling pupil, who loved reading and enjoyed her schoolwork.
What a pleasure to discuss with her – we started with looking closely at
the "Hobbit", her current book. She was anxious that she was falling
behind, having missed so much school, so I proposed some reading
assessments, which she romped through (as I expected) and which proved
she had a reading age well beyond her calendar age. Poetry too we
shared; she loved words but she did not feel well enough to write much.

She was a true scholar; in Maths she would look over her work and
spot her errors. Whatever she did, she tried to do as well as possible. She
selected her priorities for SATs, especially within Maths and Science, and
with the support of the head at Nynehead School, we worked steadily as
her varying condition would permit. As SATs approached and her
condition worsened, we decided to drop anything not immediately vital –
the French games, for example, which had given her fresh confidence in
her linguistic abilities.

It is amazing that on the days when she was unable to get to School,
she still managed to concentrate on some study. She was in and out of
hospital and I liaised with Jenny Fisher, in charge of education on the
children's unit. Jessie was determined to do her SATs and do them well.
(She did). However, there were days when her mother would ring me in
advance and ask me "just to play a game" for mental stimulation rather
than have a formal session. Jessie, lying on the sofa, would take part as

much as possible – and her favourites were word games like "Boggle" and "Anagram"; we played the latter on her birthday and she loved the challenge.

After SATs, Jessie proposed her own History project, investigating the life of one of her ancestors who was a policeman in Victorian times. She consulted all sorts of sources, sharing both the labour and the results with the rest of the family. Her mother supported these efforts in every way and shared her very considerable artistic skill, which Jessie had inherited. Throughout my time teaching Jessie, she was busy with art; a wonderful drawing of a lion now has pride of place on the sitting room wall. She loved making things; we made a cat and mouse toy on magnetic principles! But she also enjoyed looking at various works of art and discussing the styles – she made a good attempt of sketching her own bedroom as a reflection in a convex mirror, such as the one used by Van Eyck in The Arnolfini Marriage. She was always ready to try something out!

I was delighted to be invited to her confirmation in May and to witness her vows. God was with her at all times – when she put a brave face on for me on a bad day and when sharing her delight at the good times. One of the best times was her party, the day after her 11th birthday on 25th May. I felt very privileged to be able to join in such a special occasion and share the fun with all her family and friends.

It was a comfort to know that Jessie had a good summer, following the serious operation in June. When she started at Court Fields School in September, she went full-time and did not need me; I was delighted. Alas, it was not to last, by half-term the cancer and pain had returned – with a vengeance. Jessie took the decision not to continue with treatment when there was no hope and equally decided that there was no further point in formal education. For one of my last sessions we had a great time making butter sculptures but I was not to see her much more; on good days she wanted freedom but on bad ones she slept. Time was precious, so was energy, she was growing up fast, making choices most adults do not have to make. I admired her, I missed her company and she was in my thoughts and prayers. When faced now with a healthy young person, excluded and seemingly throwing life away, I think of her, how positive she tried to be; this contrast is the hardest part of my work.

Her early death was tragic but Jessie gave us all the gift of having known her. Her funeral at Nynehead was a most wonderful celebration of her life, in a church packed by people of all ages. Grief is the price we pay for love and friendship. Her spirit lives on. Thank you, Jessie, for sharing a small part of your life with me.

She inspired me, when I became president of Taunton Vale Inner

Wheel a few years later, to lead the club in some very successful fundraising for the new Children's Hospice at Charlton Farm.

- Laurian Cooper
Home Teacher for Somerset Tuition Service

My best memories are of Jessie when well, when her bubbly character would shine through, and she let her sense of humour run loose. She had an infectious laugh, and an ability to cheer others up when times were rough. She had this incredible tendency to push limits to the max – my medical mind found it hard to imagine her bouncing on the trampoline so soon after chemo or her operation, but she did it in style and proved me very wrong!

That same determination was so evident in the difficult times too – there was never a time when Jessie didn't have an opinion on something, or didn't want to face up to impossible decisions. From very early on it was clear that there was no protecting her from the awkward bits of discussions that are often reserved for the adults – eg "where do the organ donors come from?" taken to its full limits when she was only 10, and facing a possible transplant herself. That type of discussion was only a brief introduction to her inquisitive style and desire to face difficult philosophical issues head on, but unfortunately there were so many more difficult issues ahead, and none of them intended for girls of her age.

Although there were many dark days this time last year, my overwhelming feelings at this stage are of tremendous respect and admiration for Jessie. The last few months included huge amounts of fear and anger, but also incredible strength, love and determination from Jessie to all her family and her medical, nursing and other carers. I am very aware that she felt let down by the medical profession as a whole, as despite doing everything asked of her, we couldn't keep "our end of the bargain" and get rid of the her cancer. But this didn't stop her sense of humour (Embodied so graphically in her famous tee-shirt), her determination to be in charge of decisions which affected her, and her tremendous love for her family and desire to protect them from harm or pain. Inspirational, and an example to us all. I will always treasure our last good-bye.

My thoughts are with you this Christmas, which I know will be so hard this year. May you share in Jessie's strength and love for each other, and let her smile shine through.

Love Nicky
- Dr Nicky Harris 24th December 2002
Associate Specialist in Paediatric Oncology
Musgrove Park Hospital, Taunton

I met Jessica on 12th December 2000, the day she was admitted to Bristol Children's Hospital. We admit over a hundred new children a year to the hospital from the South West Region for diagnosis and treatment of cancer of one sort or another. Usually treatment is effective and often much of the child's treatment can be carried out at a General Hospital nearer their home after the initial diagnosis and starting the treatment but they do have to come to Bristol for things such as surgery and for the more complex treatment regimes.

Unfortunately Jessica had a particularly difficult form of cancer, both to diagnose and to treat and these challenges are one of the reasons I remember Jessica so well. The other reason I remember her so well was her quite outstanding personality. She was an intelligent child who took a lively interest in everything that was going on and always wished to be personally involved in discussion and decisions. Patients we treat range from new born babies up to teenagers. Obviously with the very youngest children all the discussion has to be with the family, at the other end of our age scale many teenagers "switch off" and abrogate responsibility to others. Jessica was a wonderful example of a child in the in between age group who is able to understand and take control of the complex management of their own illness. Much of the time I saw her she was extremely ill but in periods where she was less ill it was a delight to see her intelligence and sense of humour coming through.

Over two thirds of the children we treat are cured. Unfortunately Jessica came into the minority group where a cure is not possible. Health Professionals can do a number of things which may help t alleviate symptoms but the chief burden falls on the child and those close to them in managing the progressive effects of incurable cancer.

I believe that Jessica managed this phase of her illness as bravely and appropriately anyone of any age could have done. In this she was supported by her loving family.

My work is often difficult and I am helped very much by letters of thanks from children and their families when things go well and difficult diseases are cured but of course mostly by seeing those children who were once ill restored to normal life. Part of the job has to be finding a way to cope with the unsuccessful outcomes. I have to say I have discovered no easy way to do this; I find the premature death of a child just as difficult to cope with now as I did when I first encountered incurable children over thirty years ago. I have the most enormous admiration for children and families who find the strength to cope in a positive way in situations which I know I would find so difficult.

- **Mr Richard D Spicer**
Consultant Paediatric Surgeon
Bristol Royal Hospital for Children

I remember Jessica and her family well.
My first contact was from the caring medical team through emails that described the difficulties she had facing her at diagnosis and the first weeks of treatment, though her condition did improve with time and good care.
When I saw Jessica the first time, she had recovered well from these problems and was happy that further treatment could be considered. She had already forgotten the recent events and was looking forward to the future. She was confident in the medical staff and we on our side put our greatest efforts to follow her hopes. She had been expecting everything but asking little, patient in all senses of that word, calm and trusting.
Neither as a father, nor as a surgeon, can I understand the way diseases can take children away from us. I can only fight with my hands and my heart, accepting not to be able to help children always to win their battle. All of them remain in my memory. Their trust in me supports me and helps me to continue fighting for others and helps making the fight more successful next time.
Thank you Jessica.
- Professor Jean de Ville de Goyet

I met Jessica during her extremely rare illness. She made an impression which has stayed with me ever since and this has influenced my clinical approach to sick children. Jessica was extremely courageous in accepting her condition and its subsequent complications relating to the treatment. I was amazed at her willingness and kindness she showed despite having a life threatening illness. I was extremely pleased to hear of her mother's decision to publish a book relating to Jessica's illness to help others.
Finally, as a Buddhist I believe life is impermanent and perhaps Jessica understood this deep concept.
- Dr. Sunil Pullaperuma
Consultant and Honorary Senior Lecturer in Paediatric Neurodisability
St Mary's Hospital, London

I met Jessica in May 2001 in All Saint's Church, Nynehead, where I had just taken up pastoral responsibility for the church and the village community. Jessica had only days before being confirmed by The Bishop of Taunton. I did not know then how ill Jessica was, nor of the ordeal she was soon to face as she battled bravely with a very serious form of cancer.

Yet in those moments of our first meeting I was struck by this lovely young girl, standing in front of me, whose face was alight with joy. Something shone out of Jessica, something beyond delight even, as she told me she had been confirmed. She had taken this important step in faith towards the Lord Jesus whom she had chosen to follow, to trust, and to love. Without knowing the situation Jessica was facing, I knew in those moments, that I had met with someone very special, whose whole being and personality was lifted up and offered in the gift of her most wonderful, happy, and loving smile. In the months ahead when surgery and chemotherapy were to become such an intense part of Jessica's life, I never saw that smile diminish.

There are many things I'll remember, with love and gratitude for having known Jessica, but some stand out in particular and I'd like to share them now with all who read this tribute.

Christmas is a special time for us all, and of course children look forward with excitement to the parties, presents, and sheer sparkle of Christmastide. Jessica wanted to achieve one thing in particular. Although undergoing heavy anti-biotic treatment, which made her very weary – She was determined to be in St John the Baptist Parish church in Wellington at midnight on Christmas Eve to celebrate the birth of Jesus with the whole Christian Community.

As I walked up the aisle, in procession with the choir and other ministers, feeling quite hemmed in on either side by the volume of people who had come to celebrate this great festival –I saw, under a white furry hat, Jessica's lovely face beaming out at me. That smile again which brought a light to that place which no end of Christmas sparkle could have, and I rejoiced in knowing that Jessica had made it to a service which was so important to her.

After the service when other people, out of genuine courtesy, were shaking hands. Jessica gave me one of the warmest and most sincere hugs, and it touched me deeply. This brave young girl, who knew this would be her last Christmas here, yet in that knowledge was able to give out so much love to those around her.

Then there was the time when I visited her at home, unannounced. Jessica, with her Mother Kirsty, was just about to put on a face pack! She had also, that lunchtime been given a special lunch at a large hotel in

Taunton and the staff had given Jessica some delicious hand-made chocolates to take home with her. Jessica, being her generous self, offered me one of the chocolates and we laughed as we ate them about me not catching her in the face-pack. It was so good to be able to share those light-hearted moments with her and to know that when I had left the house she would put on the face pack. Doing what most young girls delight in as they begin a more mature phase of their lives. I, like any normal human being, thought as I walked to my car, if only something could be done for Jessica that would make her well again.

Sadly this was not to be for on 18 February 2002 Jessica died in Little Bridge House (Children's Hospice) in Barnstaple. This was a very sad day for all who had known and loved Jessica, and who had watched her brave battle against the cancer that would finally take her life.

I went to Little Bridge House with a colleague and Jessica's former Head Master from Nynehead School. As we were helping the family to put the funeral service together her mother handed me a poem that she had found and that she wanted me to read at the service, because she said "Jessica loved Josie" I was moved to tears. This is the poem:

A Gift from God

An Angel was sent from heaven above
A special one that would bring much love
God knew that this precious life would be short
So he looked around for a tender heart

He made his choice and the gift was sent
In what seemed like a moment, the Angel went
Leaving treasured memories, and a heart full of pain
A void, an abyss, tears followed like rain

But....

Wait just a moment, I wish you could see
The wonderful thing that's happened to me
Jesus was waiting, His arms opened wide
And He and His Angels brought me inside
Such a beautiful place that I cannot describe
A new home for me from the moment I died

I'll wait here for you, so dry up your tears
And go bravely on with your life free from fears
Know that God's near you to help and to guide

He'll never desert you, He's there by your side
So speak to him daily from inside your heart
And let him assure you, we're not really apart
(Unknown)

I have a photograph of Jessica in my special place in my house and so
I have a reminder, daily, of this beautiful young girl whose enduring
bravery was an example to all who knew her. I thank God for Jessica,
for having known her, and for all she gave to so many of us in her
short life.
With love
- Reverend Josie Harrison

J *oy of love and peace*
E *ver in our hearts*
S *pecial like a bright*
S *hining Star*
I *nto God's loving*
C *are you have been called*
A *lways in our thoughts, always loved*
Written by Monica Chapman (Auntie Mo)
- Jessica's Godmother

Memories from Grandma

You were our Angel, our Dove and our Star
Although we know just where you are
Your driving instructions that I recall
When I collected you in your last year at school
"All right Grandma, Go, Go, Go!"
This was your answer when you thought me too slow

You were too good for this turbulent time
A gift of life taken in your prime
You never spoke ill and loved every one
You had so much courage and oodles of fun
You bravely kept going with the fight you endured
Although you knew you could never be cured

You were so bold and spoke your mind
All the time so gentle and kind
We all have a mixture of sorrow and rage
Why did you leave us at such a young age?
A child so special, a child so kind
Never an evil thought in your mind

You worked so hard in your eleven years
That, inevitably were reduced to tears
The sound of your voice keeping siblings in shape
When trampolining or watching a tape
Not a moment was wasted playing Grandad at chess
Or feeding the animals, cleaning their mess

So many hobbies right from the start
Reading and writing, sewing and art
Swimming and Skating, you loved a game
We miss your enjoyment, it isn't the same
With fun loving parties, dimples and smiles
You coped with it all till you ran out of miles

Our love for you Jess, will never fade
You were our Angel so good and so brave
Nothing will ever mend the hurt felt inside
We look on you now with eternal pride
That you were taken has broken my heart
Your radiance shone brightly right from the start

We know you are safe now and out of pain
In the arms of our lord you will remain
We loved you Jess and still have tears
Remembering your diplomacy, beyond your years
With so much courage you inspire us all
To continue in life despite your call
- With love from Grandma Kodritsch xx

*I have so many memories of you, most of them happy but of course
some inevitably sad. However, the ones that always come to mind are
those of you dressing up here at our house. You especially liked the long
dresses and capes. The other thing you loved doing was playing with
the Henna beads. I clearly remember trying to get a design ironed for
you to take home.*
*Dear Jess you were so very brave and you made us feel so very humble
with your courage. I think of you up there looking after our dear little
Darcy*
'One more Angel in Heaven, One more star in the sky'
Our love always
- Auntie May & Uncle Alan XX

*It is better that I knew you and taught you for only a short time than
not at all.*
*You were and will continue to be, a credit to your family and an
example to us all*
You are in a better place now
God Bless
- Chris Moyse (P.E. Teacher)

How mature and dignified you were in French, and how good!
You would look right through me at times.
A great example to us all, I know you're at peace now
With love
- Sophie Cooke (French Teacher)

You were with us for such a short time yet you achieved so much. Your
enthusiasm, determination and sheer love of life was an inspiration to
us all.
I'm so glad we had a chance to get to know you – if only it could have
been longer.
- Chris de la Croix (Head of Year 7)

I only taught you for a short time but I shall remember you as an
enthusiastic student – always smiling.
I am glad to have known you, I learnt a lot from you.
- Lorraine Wilton (Food/ Technology Teacher)

I only had the pleasure of knowing you for a short time but I remember
your commitment to joining in all the activities each lesson. You were
enthusiastic when singing the register and "16 Tons". In group work
you helped your group to write your blues song and clearly enjoyed
rehearsing and performing it.
I can not even begin to imagine what you went through
during your illness but you can now rest in peace knowing that you
gave the very best you could during the short life you had.
God Bless
- Miss Jarvis (Music Teacher)

You were a pleasure to teach and a true star!
Bright, Bubbly and above all kind – a soothing influence on others,
your presence is missed.
My abiding memory of you (as Becky has also mentioned) was your
stunning performance of Kylie Minogue in front of 29 other students.
Few people could have carried it off – but you did it with such finesse
and your voice was so beautiful that the whole class fell silent – and
gave you spontaneous applause. That quality, was star quality – and
you had it in bucket loads!
7SK won't forget you – and neither will I
- Vicky Brown (Head of English)

I Believe....
J *ews have the right to be treated the same as us*
E *veryone in my family comes first*
S *ecrets should be kept*
S *omeone is very special*

L *ife is a precious thing to take care of*
E *veryone has the right to be respected*
I *like the taste of chocolate*
G *iving away secrets you can lose friends*
H *elping others is nice*

F *riends should be kept*
I *have the best friend ever*
R *espect for others is very important*
B *elieve in what you want*
A *lways be kind to your friends and family*
N *ever lie to your family*
K *ids should be treated with respect*
By Jessica Leigh-Firbank

You wrote this acrostic poem about your beliefs in an R.E. lesson – I
think it sums up your attitude to life better than anything I could write
here. It was a pleasure to teach you.
Rest in Peace
- Bill Revans (R.E.Teacher)

You were a box of surprises
A talent waiting to flourish
A joy to know
A pleasure to teach
You touched our lives in a unique way
It's the quality of your personality and the sweetness of your memory
that we value
We'll miss you
- Kath Sidgwick (Art Teacher)

So what do I remember most about you, Jess? In the relatively short time I knew you, you made a deep and long-lasting impression on me. I shall remember and treasure your positive outlook, your sense of fairness, your motivation and your sense of fun. I loved to hear your giggles!
I recall you coming to see me in my office to share a concern you had about a student in the Tutor group. You were worried and thought that something should be done before the student got into more trouble. You showed that you cared and I was left in no doubt that I had to do something about it!!!
I know that your visits to hospital were uncomfortable and I enjoyed my visits to see you and the conversations. We shared our views on music, your passion for pop music, and what was happening in 'Eastenders'. At one stage you turned to your Mum and with lots of giggles said, "I can't believe I'm talking about Eastenders with a Deputy Headteacher!!!"
Your visit to the Tutor group in January was very special. A time for lots of laughter and fun and for 7SK to share news, gossip and presents. I am pleased that we have that very special memory.
You were a remarkable young girl, Jess, who touched our hearts. We shall miss you.
- Gaynor Gibson
Deputy Headteacher Court Fields Community School

In your brief time in our tutor group you made a great impression!
You were voted reserve form representative and had gained over 30
merits
You had 100% attendance until you had to visit hospital more
regularly and you worried about letting the form down when you had
to stay in for treatment.
You had a tremendously unifying effect on the group bringing different
friendship groups together as you were friendly with everyone.
When I visited you in hospital you kept me entertained with
fascinating conversation and I had to drag myself away!
In your short time at Court Fields School you had a greater impact
than I could ever have imagined and you will always be part of the
tutor group.
It has been a privilege to know you
You are now at peace
- Sue McKen with love (form tutor)

I was the Headteacher of Nynehead Primary School for the whole of
Jess's time at the school. This is different from being the Head of a larger
school – Nynehead has just 2 classes so I taught the Junior class for
much of the time and got to know all the children really well. People often
said the school was like a very large family, and so it was – children of
all ages played together and the whole school could go on an outing
together in a single coach. It is sometimes implied that the bigger an
organisation is the more important or valuable it is, but I never saw it
like that. Every parent knows that each of their children is unique and
in a way, infinite – it doesn't matter if you're talking about one child, a
dozen or a thousand.

I remember that one morning Jess's skin turned yellow. We phoned her
parents, she went to the doctors', and we feared she might have hepatitis.
It was a huge shock to learn she had liver cancer. Why Jess? She was a
normal, happy child. She worked hard, got on well with her friends, was
sometimes a little disorganised. Luckily she had a good sense of humour
and could smile at herself if she got in a tangle about anything.

What emerged through her illness was an incredible determination to
lead as normal a life as possible. I can only try to imagine how she really
was feeling inside but I never saw any signs of self-pity or wanting to
take things easy. Indeed the only time I got annoyed with her was when
I learnt she had volunteered with a supply teacher to carry some things
back from the local church – she really did not want to slow down or be

different at all from the other children. Everyone's fondness of her and respect for her grew and grew. I remember she was a little sensitive after her hair fell out due to chemotherapy – then several of the boys had very short haircuts in sympathy and one took to wearing a headscarf! In the summer term of year 6 she ignored my entreaties to take it easy: she determinedly worked hard for her SATs and did very well in them too. I guess she had become very aware of what was really important in life – she didn't like people squabbling or falling out, and I believe the other children sensed this in her.

In the Autumn Jess moved on to secondary school but remained in close contact, something it was easy to do with Gemma and Stewart still at the school. We all hoped and prayed that the remission she enjoyed for a few months would last but of course it returned and spread, and the time came that Jess took the typically brave decision not to continue with invasive treatments that would ruin her quality of life and had no realistic chance of success.

I spent a long weekend in February on a leadership training programme in London. For some reason I was awake in the small hours of Monday 18 February and I was thinking about all the things in life most important to me – my family, working with children, etc. When I got home later that day I learnt that Jess had died during the night, I think at about the time I had been awake.

At school the sense of loss was deeply felt by everyone. There was no rule book to say how to navigate the coming days but it felt most important to involve all the children in what followed. They had the chance to write or draw their memories of Jess and what came out was so simple, pure and true. It felt so right when Kirsty and Jerzy decided to fill the church with balloons and make Jess's funeral a celebration of her life, so on the afternoon we closed the school and let every family decide if they wanted to come or not. Nearly everyone did. I had a strong sense of being the voice of the whole school as I read out some of the beautiful tributes written by children of all ages.

We try to make sense of the things that happen in life and Jess's o-so-early passing on is one of the very hardest. There was something rather awesome about her calmness, lack of self-pity and indeed love for others that was felt by everyone at school, adults and children alike. I can't make sense of her life being so short but I do know that she has greatly enriched my life – it was a pleasure and a privilege to have known her.

- Peter Pearson
Headteacher of Nynehead Primary School

Jess our Darling Daughter
So full of Life, yet you were taken from us
You will forever be Loved and Missed
*- **All my Love Dad x***

Dearest Jess
I remember your Smile, that glint in your eye
I never forget as the years go by
I'll always remember and cherish your love
And send hugs and kisses to heaven above
A part of me died when you left me that day
It was hard to go on, to find my way
But closing my eyes, I clearly see
Your strength and courage which inspire me
I'll love you forever and know you to be
An Angel in Heaven but a part of me
*- **My love always Mum x***

May the winds of love blow softly
From Earth to Heaven Above
Keep gently, oh so gently
In God's Eternal Love
*- **(Unknown)***

Author, Kirsty Bilski has her own website:

www.myangeltree.com

To puchase other publications please visit:

www.apexpublishing.co.uk